378 CC

EW

Getting into
Medical
School
2022 Entry

Adam Cross and Emily Lucas
26th edition

0 5 MAY 2021

trotman

Getting into guides

Getting into Art & Design Courses, 11th edition
Getting into Business & Economics Courses, 14th edition
Getting into Dental School, 12th edition
Getting into Engineering Courses, 6th edition
Getting into Law, 13th edition
Getting into Oxford & Cambridge 2022 Entry, 24th edition
Getting into Pharmacy and Pharmacology Courses, 2nd edition
Getting into Physiotherapy Courses, 10th edition
Getting into Psychology Courses, 13th edition
Getting into Veterinary School, 12th edition
How to Complete Your UCAS Application 2022 Entry, 33rd edition

Getting into Medical School

This 26th edition published in 2021 by Trotman Education, an imprint of Trotman Publishing Ltd, 21d Charles Street, Bath BA1 1HX

© Trotman Publishing Ltd 2021

Authors: Adam Cross and Emily Lucas
24th–25th edns: Adam Cross and Emily Lucas
18th–23rd edns: James Barton and Simon Horner
16th–17th edns: Simon Horner
15th edn: Simon Horner and Steven Piumatti

British Library Cataloguing in Publication Data
A catalogue record for this book is available from the British Library

ISBN 978 1 912943 42 5

Printed and bound in the UK by Ashford Colour Press Ltd.

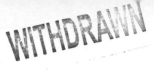

Contents

About the authors

Adam Cross is Vice Principal at MPW Birmingham and has many years' expertise in helping students gain entry onto competitive undergraduate courses, such as dentistry and medicine. He is also the current co-author of Trotman's *Getting into Dental School* guide. In addition to his careers guidance expertise, Adam also helps students with pre-admissions tests such as the University Clinical Aptitude Test (UCAT) and BioMedical Admissions Test (BMAT). Adam is a highly regarded teacher of biology and his commitment to pedagogy ensures that he keeps up to date with developments in the fields of science and teaching and learning.

Emily Lucas read medical science at the University of Birmingham before obtaining a master's degree in genomic medicine from Queen Mary, University of London. She currently holds the position of University Support Officer at MPW and helps students with their university applications, as well as supporting students with pre-admissions tests such as the University Clinical Aptitude Test (UCAT) and the BioMedical Admissions Test (BMAT). As well as teaching, Emily has maintained a research position at the University of Birmingham in the field of epigenetics. Emily also teaches biology, and is the current author of Trotman's *Getting into Law* and *Getting into Veterinary School* guides, and co-author of the *Getting into Dental School* guide.

Acknowledgements

We would like to thank MPW and Trotman Education for giving us the opportunity to produce this edition of *Getting into Medical School*. Many thanks are due to all those who have written previous editions.

We would like to thank all of the individuals who have contributed to the book, especially Dr Simon Bramhall, Camrun Shah, Pranay Ruparelia, Dr Erzsike Szabo, Usmaan Khan, Dr Sabrina Kayani, Dr Rachel Tattersall, Dr Josh Davies, Anushka Shah and Katy Glenn for their insights into applying to, studying and working in the field of medicine. In addition, we would like to thank Neelima Menon, Ebaney Ghotra, Harjan Boora and Katy Glenn for allowing us to reproduce their personal statements here as successful examples. We are extremely grateful that these individuals were willing to take time out of their busy schedules to contribute.

We would also like to thank those at UCAS, the British Medical Association and university admissions departments who have supported us by answering our questions regarding statistics and general advice.

Adam Cross and Emily Lucas
November 2020

About this book

This book is divided into 12 main chapters, which aim to cover three major obstacles that would-be doctors may face:

- getting an interview at medical school
- getting a conditional offer
- getting the right A level grades (or equivalent).

The 12 chapters discuss the following:

1. the study of medicine
2. getting work experience
3. deciding where to apply
4. the UCAS application
5. personal statements
6. the interview process
7. current issues that may come up at interview
8. results day
9. non-standard applications
10. fees and funding
11. careers opportunities
12. further information.

Chapter 1 gives information on the actual study of medicine, different teaching styles and postgraduate study, as well as possible specialisations and post-degree course options.

Chapter 2 deals with the significance of undertaking work experience and voluntary work, how to make the most of your placements and how to secure them.

Chapter 3 looks at the different aspects that you should consider when choosing a medical school.

Chapter 4 provides information on the more technical aspects of the UCAS application, with key pointers on how to use UCAS Apply and how to prepare for relevant entrance exams such as the UCAT and BMAT.

Chapter 5 gives an insight into how to write an outstanding personal statement, including how to deliver your points effectively and make your application stand out.

Chapter 6 provides advice on what to expect at the interview stage, current topics, issues you may be questioned about and how to come across as a prospective doctor.

Chapter 7 presents some key information on contemporary and topical medical issues, such as the structure of the NHS, diseases that are appearing in the media, and legal issues that have made the headlines in recent years. Knowing about medical issues is a must, particularly if you are called in for an interview.

Chapter 8 looks at the options that you have at your disposal on results day and describes the steps that you need to take if you are holding an offer or if you have been unsuccessful and have not been given an offer.

Chapter 9 is aimed primarily at overseas students and any other 'non-standard' applicants – mature students, graduates, students who have studied arts A levels and retake students (most medical schools consider non-standard applicants). The chapter also includes some advice for those who want to study medicine outside the UK, say, for example, in the US.

Chapter 10 gives some useful information regarding fees and funding for medical students, as well as bursaries and scholarships that are available, while **Chapter 11** looks at career options in medicine.

Finally, in **Chapter 12**, further information is given in terms of courses and further reading. A number of other excellent books are available on the subject of getting into medical school. The contact details of the various medical groups and universities can also be found here. After Chapter 12 a **Glossary** can be found of many of the terms used throughout the book.

The book also contains numerous case studies and examples of material that will reflect to some extent the theme being discussed at that point. We hope that you find these real-life examples illuminating.

Finally, the views expressed in this book, though informed by conversations with staff at medical schools and elsewhere, are our own, unless specifically attributed to a contributor in the text.

If you have any comments or questions arising from this book, the staff of MPW would be very happy to answer them. You can contact us at the address given below. Good luck with your application to medical school!

Adam Cross and Emily Lucas

MPW (Birmingham)
16–18 Greenfield Crescent
Edgbaston
Birmingham B15 3AU
Tel: 0121 454 9637

Introduction

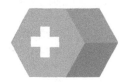

'For me, it is the constantly changing environment of working in A&E that I enjoy the most. While the patient interactions are relatively brief, the immediate impact that you have at that moment in time is massively rewarding. There is never a dull moment and it is a role that is entirely stimulating on an intellectual level, and it gives me the opportunity to channel my scientific enthusiasm in a humanistic way.'

Dr Daniel Adey

Perhaps now more than ever, at the height of a global pandemic, it is unusual for a day to pass without hearing about the NHS. In recent years, it has been the media's soft toy, often vilified, rarely championed and yet the reality is, the system is simply a victim of its own success. Its chronic underfunding has been brought to light by the Coronavirus pandemic, but it has also unified the country in its appreciation for the outstanding work conducted by its frontline staff. Over the past 50 years, the NHS has made enormous strides, and there is more than one convincing reason to confidently argue that it is better now than ever. It has become better at saving people's lives. This is enormously positive, and yet it means its failures become more transparent, as public expectation in the health-care sector is now at a level whereby people expect to be saved.

This is where you come in, as aspiring doctors, for which there will always be demand. This book is designed to provide you with much of the information required to formulate a successful application to medical school.

A realistic chance

In previous years, only around 12% of applicants for medicine were successful in gaining places. Does this mean that the remaining 88% were unsuitable? The answer, of course, is no. Many of those who are rejected are extremely strong candidates, with high grades at GCSE under their belts and personal qualities that would make them excellent doctors. Typically, there are a fixed number of medical school places available each year and so not all candidates can be successful. However, many promising applicants do not put themselves in a position whereby they can be given proper consideration, simply because they do not prepare well enough.

Ideally, your preparation should begin at least two years before you submit your application, but if you have come to the decision to apply to study medicine more recently, or if you were unaware of what steps you need to take in order to prepare a strong application, it isn't too late. Even over a relatively short period of time (a few months), you can put together a convincing application.

In 2019, UCAS reported a five-year high for students applying to study medicine, with 23,710 applicants submitting their UCAS choices by the October 15 deadline. It is thought that the increase in the number of applicants is a consequence of the increased number of medical school places that became available. UCAS received applications from 18,500 UK students, with a further 1,680 from EU students and 3,530 from international students outside of the EU. These students were battling for approximately 9,310 places available at UK medical schools.

The grades you need

Table 11 (see pages 221–224) shows that, with a few exceptions, the A level grades you need for medicine are AAA, though there are some A* offers around now. A number of medical schools, including Cambridge, Imperial College London, Oxford, King's College London, Queen Mary, Queen's University Belfast and University College London are asking for an A* grade in their entry offers going forwards. Other universities, such as Plymouth, also state that an A* grade *may* be stipulated as part of their offer. For students who are retaking their A levels, A* grades are often included in offers, such as the University of East Anglia who outline this condition as part of their resit policy.

As a general guide, candidates with qualifications other than A levels are likely to need the following:

- Scottish: AAAAB in Highers or AA in Advanced Highers to include AAAAB in Highers
- International Baccalaureate: around 34–43 points, including 7, 7, 6–6, 6, 5 at Higher level (with most including chemistry)
- European Baccalaureate: roughly 80% overall, with at least 80% in chemistry and another full option science/mathematical subject.

But there's more to it than grades ...

If getting a place to study medicine were purely a matter of achieving the right grades, medical schools would demand A*AA at A level (or equivalent) and 10 top grades at GCSE, and they would not bother to conduct interviews. However, becoming a successful doctor requires many skills, academic and otherwise, and it is the job of the admissions staff to try to identify who of the thousands of applicants are the most suitable. It would be misleading to say that anyone, with enough effort, could become a doctor, but it is important for candidates who have the potential to succeed to make the best use of their applications.

Non-standard and second-time applications

Not all successful applicants apply during their final year of A levels. Some have retaken their exams, while others have used a gap year to add substance to their UCAS application. Again, it would be wrong to say that anyone who reapplies will automatically get a place, but good candidates should not assume that rejection first time round means the end of their medical career aspirations.

Gaining a place as a retake student or as a second-time applicant is not as easy as it used to be, but candidates who can demonstrate genuine commitment alongside the right personal and academic qualities still have a good chance of success if they go about their applications in the right way. The admissions staff at the medical schools tend to be extremely helpful and, except at the busiest points in the year when they simply do not have the time, they will give advice and encouragement to suitable applicants. With this in mind, it is worth conducting your research in good time and contacting universities well before the October application deadline in order to identify the universities to which your application would be best suited.

Admissions

The medical schools make strenuous efforts to maintain fair selection procedures: UCAS applications are generally seen by more than one selector, interview panels are given strict guidelines about what they can (and cannot) ask, and most make detailed statistics available about the backgrounds of the students they interview. Above all, admissions staff will tell you that they are looking for good 'all-rounders' who can communicate effectively with others, are academically capable and are genuinely enthusiastic about medicine – if you think that this sounds like you, then read on!

Steps to prepare you for a successful medicine application

The process of applying for medicine can be challenging, so it is vital that you take all of the necessary steps required to ensure that you have an excellent chance of securing a place.

Before you apply, thoroughly research the stages of the application process and the demands of the course and career. You should aim to:

1. establish whether medicine is the right career for you

2. secure relevant work experience and voluntary placements

3. determine whether you are up to the academic challenge of getting into medicine and studying it

4. ensure that you have the appropriate qualities to make an excellent doctor

5. identify which universities you might like to study at

6. research your chosen universities to ensure that the course they offer is suitable for your own learning needs

7. ascertain the entry requirements for your chosen universities, including academic attainment and pre-admissions testing

8. identify what makes an outstanding personal statement

9. develop your interview skills

Reflections of a doctor

The words below from qualified practitioners and a first-year medical student express and reflect some of the many challenges and rewards that you may also face in your own journey to become a doctor. As with every journey, the grandest ones start with the first minuscule step.

Case study

Dr Josh Davies graduated from the University of Birmingham's graduate medicine programme in 2018. Josh's route into the field of medicine was convoluted, and aptly demonstrates the importance of perseverance when training to become a doctor.

'My path into medicine was not the most straightforward! I always had aspirations to pursue a career in medicine, but sadly fell short of getting the required grades to enter medical school straight from A levels. I also found myself in the unfortunate position of having no back-up choice and so had to make some difficult decisions about my career path. I had always gravitated towards the sciences during my A levels, with a particular affinity for human biology. This led me to look for physiology and anatomy degrees that might give me the requisite basic science background to pursue a career in medicine as a graduate. I stumbled across the Bachelor of Medical Sciences degree offered by the University of Birmingham, and I spent the next three years completing my degree and achieving a first-class degree with honours. I went on to work full time as a healthcare assistant in a busy emergency department, learning how a multidisciplinary team works and gaining some invaluable experience in interacting with patients and their loved ones. I was fortunate enough to gain a place at medical school during this time and four years later graduated as a doctor.

'My career in medicine has only just started. I currently work as a first-year foundation doctor in a busy district general hospital in the middle of Birmingham with a varied patient demographic. One of the joys of working here is the sheer variety of medical presentations you encounter. My day job is in gastroenterology and liver medicine, which involves looking after patients with conditions such as cirrhosis and inflammatory bowel disease. I am also part of the general medical on-call team. This means I see patients in A&E or the acute medical unit who have presented to hospital and need to be looked after by a medical speciality. You spend many years learning technical knowledge at medical school, and foundation training provides a fantastic opportunity to exercise that knowledge and put it into practice.

'I have changed my mind countless times about where I see my career leading, and one of the joys of medicine is the variety of careers you can pursue. There are over 100 different specialities to choose from, so there really is something for everyone. One of the earliest distinctions I think medical students make is whether they prefer surgery or medicine. I have always been a medic at heart and my first job as a doctor in a medical speciality has only reaffirmed that desire. I hope to complete my foundation years and then dual train in respiratory and intensive care medicine.

'I find the interaction with patients the most satisfying part of my job. In my opinion, medicine represents a great marriage between technical scientific knowledge and human interaction, and I really enjoy using my skills to learn a history, examine a patient and come up with a diagnosis. If you're right, that's even better!

'The NHS is at a point in its history where we have the largest number of patients presenting to emergency departments, life expectancy is at its longest and the demand on the health service often outweighs its ability to meet those needs and expectations. The NHS in many ways has become a victim of its own success, and I suppose the biggest challenge you face is trying to deal with all of the demands that working as a doctor comes with. You have to remember that you are one person, and try to get one job done at a time to the very best of your ability.

'There are several "hot topics" that are worth familiarising yourself with prior to going for interviews or considering a career in medicine. Areas such as funding for the NHS and what services we should be providing are always matters of heated debate. Privatisation of the industry is something that is already happening, and thinking about how that impacts patients and our practice is important. Finally, issues surrounding assisted suicide and end-of-life decisions are ethical dilemmas that doctors find themselves in. Having an appreciation for ethical decisions in medicine prior to your interview can be very useful.

'If my story is anything to go by, always have a back-up plan! It took me three attempts to get into medical school, but I would not change anything about my journey. I've had the pleasure of meeting some amazing people, discovered so much about myself and the kind of doctor I want to become. Medicine needs bright, enthusiastic, young learners and I wish you all the very best as you start your own journey, however that may pan out.'

Case study

Dr Sabrina Kayani studied a medical science degree at the University of Birmingham before commencing their medicine programme, from which she graduated in 2019.

'Since graduating in 2019 from medical school, I am now just over one year into my foundation training. As a Foundation Year 1, in a teaching hospital in Birmingham, I started in urology which also involved general surgical on-calls. Starting in surgery definitely meant you hit the ground running, as not only are the ward rounds going at 100 miles per hour, but more often than not, the juniors are expected to be the constant figure on the wards, as registrars and consultants are required in theatres. This meant we learnt very early on how to manage the sick patients on the wards. Of course, we escalated as appropriate when help was required, but doing a rapid assessment, performing investigations and commencing initial management became second nature – we had to keep the patients stable, until at least someone more senior was able to offer their advice on what else needed to be done.

'Following this, I entered elderly care medicine – I found myself enjoying this rotation immensely, more so than I imagined. A lot of the patients almost become long-term residents, as they get stuck while the social aspect of their discharges takes time, and you find yourself becoming attached. There are times when this can make the job difficult, but more often than not, you find it a joy to see them every day.

'I am currently a senior house officer in paediatrics; the other end of the age spectrum to my last position. I happen to be here during "back to school" season, so was expecting an onslaught of children with runny noses and coughs. Often, the whole bay can be wheezy child after wheezy child. Interestingly, similar to the dementia patients I have dealt with, children cannot always express what is wrong with them. This detective work is what makes the job interesting.

'I currently am unable to choose an area that I am interested in specialising in – I enjoyed elderly care and am finding paediatrics just as fulfilling. However, I have yet to experience my remaining placements of obstetrics and gynaecology and GP (both were also enjoyed at medical school), so I'm just going to wait and see if I can decide at the end of FY2.

'The teams I have worked with have made the job very rewarding – I have been lucky enough to work with some of the nicest people; the knowledge and advice they have imparted has been invaluable.

'However, there are some challenging aspects of the job. There are lots of days when you end up taking your work home with you – for me, this is usually thoughts about how I've cared for a patient or if I've done my best that day. It's times like this when having a good team around you helps you process your thoughts.

'Covid-19 is, without a doubt, a hot topic in medicine at the moment. When starting my foundation job, the thought of being in the middle of a pandemic within the first year did not even cross my mind. This disease is something we have learned about so quickly, but still has so many aspects we are not sure about. I remember those first few weeks, when we knew significantly less than we do now – at those times, the hierarchy that many describe in hospital medicine had all but completely disappeared. We were all on a level playing field, all not knowing what to expect.

'The (first) peak of the pandemic meant that I remained in my job in elderly care, rather than rotating on to my next placement. Covid-19 hit the elderly patients harder than we were initially expecting. The loss of patients and staff was significant. The difficult conversations I had to have with patients and their families, I do not think I would have experienced outside of this situation. Compassion and empathy had never been more important.

'My biggest tip for aspiring medics is to make sure that you really *want* a career in medicine. It is not easy and it is not glamorous. There is a lot of work to be done, and at times the system can be frustrating. However, the experiences you will have will be like no other. I cannot see myself doing anything else.'

Case study

Katy is a first-year medical student at the University of Bristol. Katy had initially opted to study English and French at the University of Warwick before deciding that she wanted to pursue a career in medicine.

'I think that medicine is a very special degree. It is so much more than just the study of the body, health and disease – you are also learning how to be a good, compassionate and competent doctor, which encompasses learning skills in consultation, anatomy, biology, ethics, behavioural and social sciences, and lots more! You are committing to a career that involves lifelong learning and gives you the opportunity to specialise in too many areas to count or to get involved in so many other aspects of healthcare, such as research or teaching. As a degree, and a future career it is very people-focused, and it allows you to put your knowledge and skills to use on a daily basis to help people – I think this is the main reason why I chose to study medicine, as I was really attracted to the idea of studying something that I was not only interested in, but that I could also visualise using my knowledge in the future to help individuals.

'Before applying, I worked part time at a GP surgery in an administrative role for a couple of months; carried out a couple of weeks' work experience in two different hospitals local to me, which gave me the opportunity to shadow a range of healthcare professionals; and worked as a domiciliary carer for a month.

'My work experience cemented my desire to study medicine; it showed me some of the benefits and the difficult realities of working in healthcare and as a doctor. Working as a carer in particular was valuable in improving my empathy and my communication skills, and gave me an insight into the day-to-day life of people living with complex health needs and disability; this experience is really beneficial for applying to study medicine as it gave me a lot of exposure to different health needs and how they are managed at home – this gave me a lot to talk about at interview as well!

'I had a slightly unusual journey into medicine. When I originally took my A levels, I studied English Literature, History and French and then went to university to study for a degree in English Literature and

French. During the university holidays, I worked part time at a GP surgery, where I discovered that I really wanted to study medicine, and work as a doctor! I left university after my first year, and studied for A levels in Biology and Chemistry in the condensed period of one year, so that I could apply to study medicine. After studying and securing my grades, I had a year out while I was applying to medical school, during which I worked as a carer and then as a healthcare assistant in a hospital – this has been really valuable experience for me, as I have now had a lot of contact with patients, and improved my communication skills and confidence.

'Starting a medicine degree in the middle of a global pandemic has made this quite a different first-year experience – at the moment, or until things settle down, all of our teaching is online and virtual, including our GP placements. Despite this, my experience so far has been amazing, I am finding the course fascinating, and it still feels immersive and interesting despite all being on a computer screen. I am looking forward to being able to attend GP placements, tutorials and lectures "in-person" hopefully sometime soon!

'I am particularly enjoying how varied the course is, and how it is so focused on patient-centred care. I am really enjoying learning about Behavioural Social Sciences – where we are learning about things such as health behaviours and the patient–doctor relationship. I am only a few weeks into the course, however and I am sure there will be so many more aspects that I enjoy in the future! However, medicine is an incredibly vast subject, and it can be easy to feel a bit overwhelmed by the huge amount of information that is out there to learn.

'I think it's too early in the course to tell what I'll want to specialise in, but I'm excited to discover different areas of medicine and find what I am particularly interested in, and may want to specialise in, in the future.

'It can be a really daunting experience applying to medical school, and it is easy to let worries about interviews and offers get you down. Remember that you are unique and have something different to offer than other applicants! Do your research, and practise answering interview questions with friends and family, but also remember that more often than not, at interview they want to see that you are enthusiastic and able to have a genuine conversation with someone, and they want to learn more about you, your experience and your values – having set answers and rehearsed responses will not help with that! I would also say to really think about which medical school will be a good fit for you – whether you would learn best from a traditional medicine course, or an integrated course with early patient contact, whether you are excited by the thought of case-based or problem-based learning – each course is unique so it's important to do your research, and this will also help with answering questions at interview as well.'

1 | Studying medicine

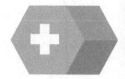

This chapter mainly discusses studying medicine as an undergraduate course. For information on postgraduate courses, see the section entitled 'Postgraduate courses' on page 25.

Medical courses are carefully planned by the General Medical Council (GMC) to give students a wide range of academic and practical experience, which will lead to final qualification as a doctor. The main difference between medical schools is the method of teaching. At the end of the five-year course, students will – if they have met the high academic standards demanded – be awarded a Bachelor of Medicine or Bachelor of Medicine and Surgery (referred to as an MB or an MBBS, respectively). Many doctors come out with an MBChB – it all depends on which medical school you go to. As with dentistry, the ChB, i.e. Honours, is largely an honorary title. The MB is the Bachelor of Medicine while the ChB is the Bachelor of Surgery from the Latin *Baccalaureus Chirurgiae*.

It is well worth noting that, at this stage, doctors are graduates and have yet to do (if they so wish) a postgraduate doctoral degree such as a PhD. So they are, in the academic and philosophic sense, not doctors. However, when doctors specialise, it is then necessary to have a postgraduate doctoral degree.

Teaching styles

The structure of all medical courses is similar, with most institutions offering two years of pre-clinical studies followed by three years of clinical studies. However, schools differ in the ways in which they deliver the material, so it is very important to get hold of, and thoroughly read, the latest prospectuses of each university to which you are thinking of applying.

Medical courses can be classified as either traditional, problem-based learning (PBL), case-based learning (CBL) or integrated. The table opposite shows a list of the medical schools in the UK along with the teaching style they practise.

Table 1 Teaching styles

Medical school	Teaching style
University of Aberdeen	Integrated
Anglia Ruskin University	Integrated
Aston University	Integrated
Barts and The London School of Medicine and Dentistry (Queen Mary University of London)	PBL
University of Birmingham	Integrated (including CBL)
Brighton and Sussex Medical School	Integrated
University of Bristol	Integrated
University of Buckingham	Integrated
University of Cambridge	Traditional
Cardiff University	PBL and CBL
University of Central Lancashire	Integrated
University of Dundee	Integrated
University of East Anglia	Integrated
University of Edinburgh	Integrated
University of Exeter	Integrated
University of Glasgow	Integrated (including CBL)
Hull York Medical School	PBL
Imperial College London	Integrated
Keele University	Integrated
King's College London	Integrated
Lancaster University	PBL
University of Leeds	Integrated
University of Leicester	Integrated
University of Liverpool	Integrated (including CBL)
University of Manchester	PBL
Newcastle University	Integrated
University of Nottingham	Integrated
University of Oxford	Traditional
University of Plymouth	PBL
Queen's University Belfast	Traditional
University of St Andrews	Integrated
St George's, University of London	Integrated
University of Sheffield	Integrated
University of Southampton	Integrated
University of Sunderland	PBL
University College London	Integrated
Swansea University	Integrated
University of Warwick	Integrated

Traditional courses

This is the more long-established, lecture-based style, using didactic methods such as lectures as a means of delivering the information.

Generally, they have a structure that consists of two or three years of taught theory, followed by two to three years of clinical training. It has to be said that these courses are a rarity today and are limited to establishments such as Cambridge, Oxford and Queen's University, Belfast, where there is a definite pre-clinical/clinical divide and the pre-clinical years are taught very rigidly in subjects.

TIP!

Find out more details about these traditional-based learning courses by going to the websites for the following medical schools:

- University of Oxford: www.medsci.ox.ac.uk
- University of Cambridge: www.medschl.cam.ac.uk
- Queen's University Belfast: www.qub.ac.uk/schools/mdbs

Course structure: Cambridge (Traditional)

Cambridge's medicine courses are intellectually stimulating and professionally challenging. They provide rigorous training in the medical sciences, while equipping students with the communication, interpersonal and clinical skills required by today's doctors.

Years 1, 2 & 3

As is typically the case with traditionally taught courses, at Cambridge, students are taught the medical sciences for the first three years, which are referred to as pre-clinical studies.

Pre-clinical studies involve around 20–25 timetabled hours per week, which includes taught lectures, practical classes (such as dissections) and supervisions.

In years 1 and 2, the main academic areas covered include Functional Architecture of the Body, Homeostasis, Molecules in Medical Science, Biology of Disease, Mechanisms of Drug Action, Neurobiology and Human Behaviour and Human Reproduction. These are designed to give you an excellent foundation in medical sciences.

You will also study a clinical strand, including an Introduction to the Scientific Basis of Medicine, Social Context of Health and Illness and Preparing for Patients. While the main focus is academic during this period of the degree, the Preparing for Patients Module eases into the clinical aspects of medicine through patient interaction in a GP surgery in year 1, a hospital setting in year 2 and through visiting community-based health-related agencies in year 3.

The third year of the course allows you to specialise in an alternative subject – a process known as intercalation. Students can choose from a wide variety of subjects, such as pathology, physiology, zoology, psychology and natural sciences, or even a subject that is entirely distinct from medicine, such as anthropology, management studies or philosophy.

Upon successful completion of the first three years, you will be awarded a BA degree in your chosen subject.

Years 4, 5 & 6

The subsequent three years of a Cambridge medicine course involve learning predominantly in clinical settings, such as GP surgeries and outpatient clinics. By this point, you will be thoroughly equipped with medical knowledge, and therefore the clinical component of the course provides a crucial opportunity to develop bedside skills. These clinical sessions are supported by seminars, tutorials and discussion groups.

Clinical studies are based at the Cambridge Biomedical Campus and Cambridge University Hospitals NHS Foundation Trust, as well as a variety of other regional NHS hospitals throughout the East of England and general practices in Cambridge.

The clinical studies aim to enhance your biomedical knowledge while allowing you to hone your practical skills and attitudes required to practise clinical medicine. Each of the three years has its own focus: year 4 – core clinical practice, year 5 – specialist clinical practice, and year 6 – applied clinical practice. Each of these is based around several major themes, including communication skills, patient investigation and practical procedures; therapeutics and patient management; core science, pathology and clinical problems; evaluation and research and professionalism and patient safety.

In addition, you will also have weekly clinical supervisions. These small group sessions with junior doctors are designed to assist with the further development of your clinical skills.

After successful completion of the clinical years, you will be awarded the Bachelor of Medicine and the Bachelor of Surgery degree (MB, BChir) in addition to your BA degree.

Assessment

Assessment is continuous throughout all six years, and progress is reviewed weekly and termly by college supervisors. Formal assessments comprise written and practical examinations, coursework submission and clinical assessments. Only upon successful completion of these tasks can you progress with the course.

Problem-based learning (PBL)

The PBL course, commended by the GMC, was pioneered by medical schools such as Liverpool (which now offers an integrated course) and Manchester and subsequently taken up by a number of other medical schools such as Plymouth and Hull York. The course is taught with a patient-oriented approach. From year 1 onwards, students are heavily involved in clinical scenarios, with the focus on the student to demonstrate self-motivation and proactive, self-directed learning, both independently and as part of a small group. This type of teaching and learning is designed to get away from the previous traditional 'spoon-fed' approach; therefore, those who are used to the spoon feeding of information may take some time to adjust.

It is common now for medical schools to utilise PBL to varying levels. Some will use PBL sessions as a predominant learning tool, supplemented by lectures, whereas others will utilise them around taught content periodically.

A typical PBL session involves dissecting a case study, or 'problem', as part of a small group. Once you have been presented with this information, it is down to your group to decide what you will need to learn to handle the situation before going away and discovering it for yourselves, and then feeding back to your group coordinator. The idea is that you acquire knowledge through research-based problem solving, rather than being taught directly.

Studying at Peninsula Medical School, University of Plymouth

Students benefit from close relationships with several NHS hospital partners, where they practise their clinical and communication skills in the safe setting of Plymouth's Clinical Skills Resource Centre (CSRC). The CSRC features specially designed replicas of hospital wards and emergency rooms, with high specification patient-simulators. You will also learn from real patients from the outset, with clinical placements starting in the first two weeks of year one.

Years 1 & 2

In the first two years, students learn the core scientific foundations of medicine within a clinical context. In the first year, the curriculum is structured around the human life cycle, so in the first year, human physical and psychological development from conception to old age are studied. Students will learn from real-life clinical case studies and experience healthcare in a range of community settings, meeting patients and service users, and learning from health and social care professionals.

In the second year, the human life cycle is revisited, this time with an emphasis on disease, pathological processes and the human and social impact of illness and disease. Students undertake a series of placements in a single general practice, enabling them to learn about long-term health issues and see teamwork in action.

The modules covered over these two years include Medical Knowledge, Clinical and Communication Skills, Personal Development and Professionalism and a Student-Selected Component.

Years 3 & 4

In their third and fourth years, students will learn more about clinical practice and spend more time in a patient-centred learning environment. Completing a series of hospital and general practice-based community placements, students will gain valuable experience in a wide range of clinical settings and see first-hand how the NHS works as a team to deliver patient care.

Year 3 focuses on three Pathways of Care: Acute Care, Ward Care and Integrated Ambulatory Care.

In their fourth year, students will continue working and learning in hospital and general practice settings, further developing their communication, clinical, problem-solving and analytical skills. The three Pathways of Care continue in year four with a focus on Acute Care, Palliative Care, Oncology and Continuing Care.

Year 5

Students will now be in a position to apply the knowledge, skills and confidence they have acquired over the first four years by working 'on the job', as part of a healthcare team in action, based in either Derriford or Torbay hospital. Students become more assured when dealing with clinical situations, and develop an in-depth understanding of the principles of practice in the NHS. Supplementing their independent learning with a portfolio of indicative presentations, students will also have the opportunity to do an elective in a different social or cultural context.

Source: www.plymouth.ac.uk/courses/undergraduate/bmbs-bachelor-of-medicine-bachelor-of-surgery. Reprinted with the kind permission of the Peninsula Medical School, University of Plymouth.

PBL example

The Peninsula Medical School at the University of Plymouth follows an eight-step process, built on the literature and the school's own experience of how students learn in its setting. The eight steps are designed to develop your learning skills to ensure you are prepared for the clinical environment, where you will be faced with many new and unfamiliar situations. In doing so, PBL will help prepare you for life as a foundation doctor. The curriculum follows the life cycle, and PBL cases build in complexity to allow you to integrate and consolidate your understanding of the topics and concepts introduced in other parts of the course. Each PBL case lasts for two weeks and includes three two-hour sessions and follows an unfolding case. In PBL you will draw on your learning from other parts of the course, including small-group and lecture-style components. The final PBL session allows you to consolidate new learning and apply what you have learned to new patient scenarios.

The key learning outcomes for PBL at Peninsula Medical School include the development of transferable learning skills required for lifelong learning and applicable to your life and career as a doctor, including:

- critical thinking
- understanding uncertainty
- working with complexity
- being comfortable with the limits of knowledge
- team working.

A typical example of a case scenario would be:

Mr Ted Bryce is a fifty-eight year-old man who comes to see you (his GP), because he has been having trouble sleeping for a few months and would like some sleeping tablets.

You ask him some questions to try to find out about his insomnia and you discover: he has four children, two of whom are still at school; he works for a local engineering company, which is threatened with closure, and he feels stressed that he might lose his job and will not be able to feed his family and his house might be repossessed.

You look on the computer at his medical records and discover that he was put on medication to treat high blood pressure two years ago, but that he hasn't requested a repeat prescription for almost a year.

You check his blood pressure and find that it is a bit high.

Figure 1 Process

- Read the scenario <u>and</u>
- Ensure everybody understands the language used

- Brainstorm the issues raised by the case
- Group them according to main themes

- Determine students' prior knowledge and understanding of each of the issues
- Develop a concept map

- Identify gaps in knowledge and understanding
- Develop 'SMART' questions that promote understanding and contextualisation

- Research questions as individuals or in groups during personal study time

- Report findings to the group
- Discuss difficult concepts
- Add new learning to the concept map of the case

- Consider new learning within the context of the case
- Think about how these might apply to similar/different cases e.g. what if...? questions

- Reflect on how the group and individual members performed within the group
- Feed back what went well and what could be improved

To work through this scenario, your group will identify the main issues from the case and group them into themes. You will then consider what you already know (activate prior knowledge), using concept maps (see Figure 2).

Figure 2 Concept maps

1) identify the issues

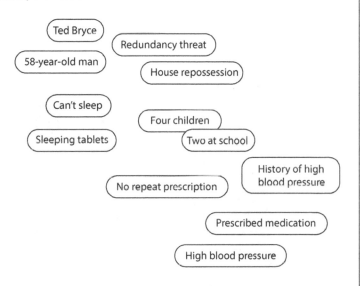

2) Group into themes

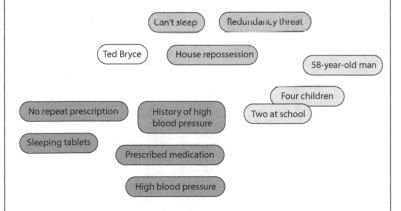

This process will also help you recognise what you don't know and set questions to develop your understanding e.g.
1. Why does narrowing of the arteries cause blood pressure to go up?
2. How do arteries become narrower?
3. How is fluid volume controlled in the body?
4. Why do people become stressed?
5. What can doctors do to help people manage stress?

6. How does stress affect sleep?
7. Why don't people take their medication?
8. How can we manage screening of all the people in the local area with high blood pressure?

Some of the issues raised will be addressed in some of the other learning sessions and some will require you to do some research, or look back at things you have done earlier in the year. The main aim is to get you thinking like a doctor and working out what you would need to know in order to help the patient and the wider population.

3) Activate prior knowledge

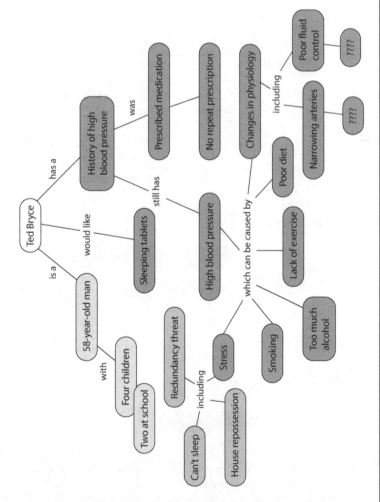

With thanks to Dr Kerry Gilbert, University of Plymouth – Lead for PBL.
Reprinted with the kind permission of the Peninsula Medical School,
University of Plymouth.

1 | Studying medicine

Integrated courses

Integrated courses are those where basic medical sciences are taught concurrently with clinical studies. Thus, this style is a compromise between a traditional course and a PBL course and, currently, is the most common type of medical course. Although these courses have patient contact from the start, there is huge variation in the amount of contact from school to school. In Year 1, contact is quite often limited to local community visits, with the amount of patient contact increasing as the years progress. In any case, most students are quite happy with having only limited contact with patients in the first year, as they feel that at this point they do not have a sufficient clinical knowledge base to approach patients on the wards.

With clinical training taking place alongside taught theory, students are able to develop both their knowledge and clinical aptitude side by side. It is an approach that is thoroughly endorsed by the General Medical Coun cil and is therefore adopted by a large number of universities.

Studying at the University of Exeter Medical School (integrated)

Throughout the duration of the medicine programme at the University of Exeter, students will study in a variety of clinical locations across the South West: in hospitals, general practice and the wider health community.

The core curriculum delivers the essential knowledge and skills for your role as a newly qualified doctor while allowing you a degree of freedom in choosing a wide range of Student Selected Special Study Units that amount to approximately one-third of the programme. Exposure to the clinical environment begins in the first week and hands-on community experience increases throughout the degree. The programme integrates medical science and clinical skills so that your academic learning is applied to clinical practice throughout the five years.

Years 1 & 2

For the first two years, students will be based at the St Luke's Campus, Exeter, and will experience university life to the full. The curriculum in the first two years is based on integrated system-based patient cases with emphasis on acquiring core knowledge of biomedical, psychological, sociological and population health aspects of medicine, and relating this to medical scenarios.

These two years lay the scientific foundations for study in subsequent years, ensuring that you learn within a clinical context. The programme reflects our belief that doctors need to adopt a socially accountable approach to their work and to understand the human and societal impact of disease, as well as the community-wide context of contemporary healthcare provision.

Years 3 & 4

The third and fourth years of the curriculum are delivered in locations across the South West. You will be based at either the Wonford site at the Royal Devon and Exeter Foundation Trust in Exeter, or at the Royal Cornwall Hospital in Truro. You will rotate through a series of hospital and community placements which provide extensive experience of a wide range of clinical settings. Your learning is centred on patients and will continue to develop your problem-solving skills and increase your experience with the widest possible array of clinical scenarios.

Year 5

In your fifth year, you will learn the job of medicine and start to develop your understanding of principles of practice in the NHS. You will undertake a series of apprenticeship attachments in hospitals across the South West, including Exeter, Truro, Barnstaple and Torbay, as well as in general practice.

At this stage, you will have developed the personal and learning skills required to analyse and evaluate patients' conditions and to suggest forms of clinical management. You will also take a Student-Selected Elective which may involve clinical or research placements, or a combination of both. Many students take this opportunity to see the practice of medicine in another part of the world (see below for more details).

The emphasis is on the practical implementation of what you have learnt and is your final preparation for medical practice. You will experience working as part of a healthcare team in the clinical environment. Your independent learning is supplemented by a portfolio of 'indicative presentations', which encourages you to continue integrating your scientific and clinical knowledge. These presentations expand and depend on the knowledge and skills you have developed in years three and four. Receiving histories from patients and performing clinical examinations will by now be very familiar to you. You will also be developing your analytical skills in interpreting diagnostic tests and initiating management plans.

Foundation Year

At the end of the undergraduate programme you will receive your BMBS degree, which is a primary medical qualification (PMQ). This entitles you to provisional registration with the General Medical Council. Provisionally registered doctors can only practise in approved Foundation Year 1 posts: the law does not allow provisionally registered doctors to undertake any other type of work. To obtain a Foundation Year 1 post, you will need to apply during the final year of your undergraduate degree through the UK Foundation Programme Office Selection scheme, which allocates these posts to graduates on a competitive basis.

Intercalated degree

An intercalated degree provides the opportunity to explore another dis-cipline at degree level, bringing added breadth and depth to your study. The opportunity to intercalate is offered to the highest performing stu-dents based on assessments during the third year.

Successful applicants join the final year of an existing BA or BSc degree at the University of Exeter; some postgraduate programmes are also available. A wide range of potential options are available, including Applied Health Services Research, Medical Sciences, Neuro-science, Pharmacology and Therapeutics, Human Genomics, Environ-ment and Human Health, Biosciences, Genomic Medicine, Clinical Education, Medical Humanities, Bioarchaeology, Psychology, Sport and Exercise Science and Flexible Honours.

Although intercalation means an extra year of study, it can enhance the undergraduate experience by providing additional specialist knowledge and transferable skills which can be a real asset in your future and professional life.

Electives

The electives form a very important part of the curriculum, enabling you to experience medicine in an entirely new environment, both socially and culturally. Electives may involve clinical or research placements, or a combination of both. Many students take this opportunity to see the practice of medicine in another part of the world, for example, by explor-ing the delivery of clinical care in developing countries, through place-ments in mission or government hospitals. Other students arrange elective placements within the South West or other parts of the UK. There are few restrictions on what you might wish to do, provided this is clearly set out in the context of agreed learning objectives.

Source: www.exeter.ac.uk/undergraduate/degrees/medicine/
medicine/#Programme-structure. Reprinted with the kind permission of the
University of Exeter Medical School.

Case-based learning

This is not the same as problem-based learning, though its ideals are similar. Unlike PBL, which is focused on problem-based scenarios, case-based learning looks at case studies within a clinical environment. It is actually quite a common route for a lot of international medical schools, and has more recently been implemented by a number of UK medical schools such as Cardiff University. In addition, the University of Glasgow and the University of Liverpool have integrated the CBL approach into their curriculum to some extent. It is a popular way of learning, with a US poll among 286 students and 31 faculties displaying an 89% preference for the CBL teaching methods.

The style of teaching will be in small groups and utilises clinical cases to elicit interest and discussion in a specific part of the course curriculum. Within these sessions, activities will be carried out with a plenary session at the end for students to share their experiences and discuss the application of them in the future.

It is expected this type of learning will become more popular in the UK sooner rather than later, with more universities starting to use this style of teaching.

Case-based learning at the University of Warwick

Case-based learning (CBL) is at the core of the MBChB curriculum and is integrated across all four years of the programme. CBL is a learner-centred method of teaching and learning that we regard as 'directed discovery'. It identifies what is essential to know about a patient case while encouraging students, individually and in small groups, to take an active role in identifying what they need to learn and how they can learn it. CBL also acknowledges that students have existing knowledge and experience which they can draw upon, including contributions to group work.

The University of Warwick has adopted CBL to support students in:

- integrating learning across the biomedical, social and clinical sciences
- applying this learning to medical practice, including in the development of clinical reasoning and problem-solving skills
- developing team working, communication and professional skills
- incorporating and building upon prior knowledge and experience
- developing skills for self-directed learning.

Source: https://warwick.ac.uk/fac/sci/med/study/ugr/courseinfo/structure/elements/cbl. Reprinted with the kind permission of the University of Warwick.

Intercalated degrees

Students who perform well in the examinations at the end of their pre-clinical studies (year 2 or 3) often take up the opportunity to complete an intercalated degree. An intercalated degree gives you the opportunity to incorporate a further degree (BSc or BA) into your medical course. This is normally a one-year project, during which students have the opportunity to investigate a chosen topic in much more depth, producing a final written thesis before rejoining the main course. Usually, a range of degrees are available to choose from, such as those from the traditional sciences, e.g. biochemistry, anatomy, physiology, or in topics as different as medical law, ethics, journalism or history of medicine.

One of the most popular choices for intercalation is biomedical or clinical science. As these are research-based degrees, they provide the opportunity for medical students to enhance their scientific knowledge of an area of interest, such as neuroscience or reproductive biology, as content is often covered at a deeper level than on a medicine degree. It also gives medical students an opportunity to participate in medical research and, in some cases, may even provide a chance to secure publications.

Why intercalate?

- It gives you the chance to study a particular subject in depth.
- It gives you the chance to be involved in research or lab work, particularly if you are interested in research later on.
- It gives you an advantage over other candidates if you later decide to specialise; for example, intercalating in anatomy would be useful if you wish to pursue a career in surgery.

Why not intercalate?

If you're not interested in studying beyond a medical degree and practising as a doctor, then you might decline the opportunity to intercalate. Intercalating will increase the number of years that you end up studying, and there is an additional cost associated with this too.

The following is an example of King's College London's (KCL) intercalated degree offering. It is a one-year BSc programme giving students an option to study related subjects in more detail. This programme is taken after the second, third or fourth year of study and is signposted to anyone who is looking to work in medical research after they have completed their course.

Intercalated example

King's College London offers one of the broader programmes at university, including:

- Anatomy, Developmental and Human Biology
- Endocrinology: Clinical and Molecular
- Global Ageing, Health and Policy
- Global Health
- Imaging Sciences
- Infectious Diseases and Immunobiology
- Medical Genetics
- Neuroscience
- Pharmacology
- Physiology

- Primary Care
- Psychology
- Regenerative Medicine & Innovation Technology
- Women's Health.

The list is an example as of October 2019. Please note that the intercalated courses available are subject to change at any time, and ensure to check the university website (www.kcl.ac.uk) for the most up-to-date information.

Source: www.kcl.ac.uk/study/subject-areas/intercalated/
intercalated-bsc-courses.
Reprinted with kind permission from King's College London.

TIP!

Websites with further information about intercalated degrees:

- www.intercalate.co.uk
- www.smd.qmul.ac.uk/undergraduate/intercalated (Barts and The London School of Medicine and Dentistry)
- www.kcl.ac.uk/study/subject-areas/intercalated/intercalated-bsc-courses.aspx (King's College London)
- www.bma.org.uk/advice-and-support/studying-medicine/becoming-a-doctor/intercalated-degrees (British Medical Association)
- www.liverpool.ac.uk/medicine/study-with-us/intercalation (University of Liverpool School of Medicine)

Taking an elective

Towards the end of the course there is often the opportunity to take an elective study period, usually for two months, when students are expected to undertake a short project but are free to travel to any hospital or clinic in the world that is approved by their university. This gives you the opportunity to practise medicine anywhere in the world during your clinical years. For example, electives range from running clinics in developing countries to accompanying flying doctors in Australia. Students see this as an opportunity to do some travelling and visit exotic locations far from home before they qualify. You can also opt to do an elective at home. If you want to know more about this, go to www.worktheworld.co.uk.

It is worth noting that, at the time of writing, many electives have been negatively impacted by the Coronavirus pandemic and it is likely to have an effect on subsequent years, beyond the initial waves of infection. Medical schools will take an individualised approach to ensuring that medical students do not lose out on clinical learning time, which may mean that there is reduced flexibility in terms of options. Electives are likely to differ for several years in that they are anticipated to take place locally and for a shorter duration.

As you will see from the example course descriptions, all medical school courses cover the same essential information but can vary widely in their teaching styles; this is an important point to consider when choosing which course to apply to. Chapter 2 has further guidance on what to consider when choosing your university and course.

Postgraduate courses

There is a huge variety of opportunities and courses for further postgraduate education and training in medicine. This reflects the array of possible areas for specialisation. Medical schools and hospitals run a wide range of postgraduate programmes, which include further clinical and non-clinical training and research degree programmes.

Advice and guidance are available from the Royal College of Physicians (RCP) (www.rcplondon.ac.uk) and the individual universities. As before, you will need to check the prospectuses of individual universities for the most up-to-date information.

Examples of postgraduate courses

The following postgraduate courses are offered by the University of Nottingham.

- Applied Sport and Exercise Medicine (MSc)
- Assisted Reproduction Technology (MMedSci)
- Cancer Immunology and Biotechnology (MSc)
- Health Psychology (MSc/PhD)
- Management Psychology (MSc)
- Master of Public Health (MPH)
- Master of Public Health (Global Health) (MPH)
- Medical Education (MMedSci/PGDip/PGCert)
- Mental Health: Research and Practice (MSc/PGDip/PGCert)
- Occupational Psychology (MSc/PGDip)
- Oncology (MSc)
- Rehabilitation Psychology (MSc)
- Sports and Exercise Medicine (MSc)
- Stem Cell Technology and Regenerative Medicine (MSc)
- Work and Organisational Psychology (MSc/PGDip)
- Workplace Health and Wellbeing (Distance E-Learning MSc).

Source: www.nottingham.ac.uk.
Reprinted with the kind permission of the University of Nottingham.

Case study

Dr Rachel Tattersall is a junior doctor who graduated from the University of Warwick's graduate-entry medicine programme. She is now working as a second-year foundation (FY2) doctor.

'When studying for my A levels, I received a conditional offer of a place for medicine at the University of Leicester. Unfortunately, though, I fell short of the entry requirements as I underperformed in maths, so I opted to take a gap year to decide what to do next. After my gap year, I completed an undergraduate degree in medical science at the University of Birmingham. I was fortunate enough to get an offer for graduate-entry medicine at the University of Warwick in my final year at Birmingham and started the programme the following September.

'At the moment, I am working as an FY2 doctor in Cornwall which I love. My FY1 jobs were paediatrics, A&E and stroke medicine. My FY2 jobs are general surgery, acute medicine and general practice. At this stage, paediatrics and emergency medicine are my main interests. I really enjoyed both my FY1 rotations in these areas and have enjoyed attending our regular "Tackling Trauma" meetings where a trauma case is discussed to help improve our service. Based on my experiences so far, I am planning on applying to paediatrics and possibly specialising in paediatric emergency medicine.

'My current place of work is very busy but I really enjoy working here. As the only hospital in Cornwall, it covers a wide area with lots of remote places. It also gets especially busy in the summer with holiday-makers, so along with winter pressures you don't get any relief from May through to March! It can calm down in April, but not for long! You get to see a really interesting mix of patients and quite a lot of trauma cases before they are transferred to a tertiary hospital. It's a small enough hospital that it feels friendly and supportive but large enough that you get a good experience and can get involved.

'Feeling like you are helping people and making a difference is a real highlight of the job. You don't always get to change a patient's outcome or see them get home, but those patients who you can make smile and feel a bit better make it all worthwhile. I enjoy meeting a mix of people, both colleagues and patients, and working in a team. I also enjoy the fact that you are always learning and like the problem-solving element when working through a patient's diagnosis – it feels great when you get it right and can help!

'Alternatively, dealing with difficult patients and their relatives is really hard. When someone has a go at you and complains, it can be difficult to stay positive and keep going, but you just have to remind yourself that not everyone is like that. It is also challenging when you can't help "cure" a patient and you have to break the news to them that all we can do is keep them comfortable or help with their symptoms. Unfortunately you cannot fix everyone, but you can still make a big difference.

'I would say the "hot topics" that I have been aware of include the move to electronic systems (we have electronic prescribing, observations and handovers here), the increase in interventional radiology and therefore the change in surgery and antibiotic stewardship. While they might sound like relatively small changes, they have the potential to really transform the way that small hospitals are run.

'If you want to do medicine, don't give up if it doesn't happen straight away or you mess up an A level! You have your whole working life ahead of you and it's never too late to apply. I really enjoyed my undergraduate degree and learnt a lot. I also found that I was much more ready and prepared to start work by being a bit older. I would also say that if you have fully explored what working as a doctor is like and have realistic expectations then you won't be surprised when you start work and will love it.'

2 | Work experience

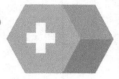

Securing a formal work experience placement is not always a prerequisite for most medical schools. However, undertaking work experience will undoubtedly bolster your application, while giving you an opportunity to reflect carefully on your decision to apply for medicine.

Why is work experience important?

Conducting work experience is typically an important part of your application: in doing work experience, you will be able to use your insights to communicate what it is about medicine that makes you want to pursue a career in the field, while being able to reflect on the less glamorous aspects of the job. It will also give you the opportunity to discuss your interests with doctors, which will allow you to garner a great deal of information about their working lives.

With this in mind, it is worth having these conversations with your own doctors, or even family and friends who work in the field of medicine. You could ask them about their time studying medicine at university and about the career options and prospects for those graduating in the field. Similarly, it is worth asking what their thoughts are on current issues and affairs in medicine and within the NHS. Remember to ask about the negative aspects as well as the positive; practising doctors are best placed to give you an accurate and honest answer.

There is no question that obtaining medical work experience can be difficult, so it is useful to get your applications in to local GP surgeries and hospitals in good time, as often, there are extended waiting lists. It is worth asking your school for support with obtaining work experience, as careers departments may have contacts that you are able to utilise.

Most work experience placements will involve shadowing a doctor. This is useful for a number of reasons:

- it will help you in determining whether you really want to be a doctor
- it will demonstrate your commitment to studying medicine
- you will be able to gain an insight into the varying nature of a doctor's working day, as well as their roles and responsibilities
- it will provide invaluable opportunities to discuss your interests in medicine

- if you make a good impression, you may be able to obtain a reference which your teacher can use to support your application.

How to arrange work experience

In some cases, your school will be able to support you by helping to organise work experience in the field of medicine, as they may have connections with local GP surgeries or hospitals. However, it is likely that only one work experience placement will be available through this route, so at some point in the process, you will need to show some initiative and organise some yourself.

Where possible, you can try and utilise any contacts that your friends and family might have. The alternative approach is to contact local GP practices and hospitals to discuss the possibility of undertaking a placement.

To obtain a work experience placement, you should:

- research local practices or hospitals
- write a formal letter or email
- contact the appropriate department to identify the name of the person who will receive your letter – in hospitals, there is likely to be a dedicated individual in each area or ward that deals with these requests, and you will want to make a good impression
- ask a teacher at your school whether they are happy to be your referee.

In addition, it is worth trying to secure placements in a medical environment, even if the role itself is not directly related to healthcare. Working on the reception desk in a GP surgery, for example, will still involve contact with patients and healthcare professionals, and can provide a valuable insight into their varying roles.

Example of a work experience request letter

Dear Mr Smith (*make sure that you contact the surgery/hospital directly and address the letter/email appropriately*)

I would be very interested in applying for some work experience at this hospital, and wondered whether any such opportunity might be available. I am currently in Year 12, studying for A levels in biology, chemistry and history, and would relish the chance to gain some practical experience during the forthcoming summer break.

I wondered whether it might be possible to meet with a doctor from your department to discuss the profession, and then perhaps spend a period of time shadowing one of your colleagues so that I am able to obtain some first-hand experience.

If you require a reference, please contact my form tutor, Mr Jones, on mrjones@teacher.ac.uk.

Please do not hesitate to contact me if you require any further information or would like me to come to your office to meet you in person.

I look forward to hearing from you.

Yours sincerely,

Robert Smith

Things to look out for during your placement

As discussed, securing a work experience placement can be difficult, so it is crucial that you make the most of it while you are there. It will allow you to improve your understanding of medicine as a career, and will provide plenty of opportunities for you to reflect on the field for discussion later in your application. As such, you should pay close attention to what is going on around you.

You could make a good impression by:

- behaving impeccably at all times
- dressing formally
- asking questions to improve your understanding of a situation (however, you should also be aware of your surroundings; it may be insensitive to ask about a disease in front of a patient, or to ask complex questions while a doctor is carrying out a procedure)
- offering to help with routine tasks
- showing an interest in things that are going on around you.

There are several things that you should keep an eye out for when undertaking your work experience placement.

- **The attributes of a doctor.** Identify the key characteristics that they display, and most importantly, when they utilise them. In doing so, you will be able to identify the traits that you may need to develop.
- **How a doctor interacts with patients.** A key aspect of medicine is communication and, as discussed later in the book, it is likely to form a part of your application or be discussed at interview. You should pay close attention to how doctors deal with patients, including how they deliver news.
- **The tasks that the doctor carries out.** Again, this will give you an opportunity to see what kind of practical skills you might need to develop. It will give you an insight into the kind of things you might need to do yourself in several years' time.

- **The interventions carried out.** During your placement, you might see doctors prescribing drugs, conducting surgery or carrying out other medical procedures. Where necessary, you should consider asking what they are, and why they are being used. While you are not expected to understand the technical nature of medicine before studying it, these observations will enhance your understanding of the roles of a doctor from preventative to curative medicine.
- **The importance of a multidisciplinary team.** While your primary focus will probably be on the doctors, they do not function alone and rely heavily on other healthcare professionals, such as nurses, receptionists and administrators. If possible, you should also try and talk to these individuals, as it is important to develop your understanding of how a doctor is supported in their work.

You might also want to consider keeping a diary to write down what you see being done. This will allow you to conduct the most important aspect of carrying out work experience – reflection. At the time, you may think that you will remember what you saw, but it could be a long time between the work experience and an interview, and you will almost certainly forget vital details. Very often, applicants are asked at interview to expand on something interesting on their UCAS application. For example:

> **Interviewer:** I see that you observed doctors treating a case of dystonia. What was that like?
>
> **Candidate:** Er.
>
> **Interviewer:** What exactly is dystonia? How was the patient treated?
>
> **Candidate:** Um.

Don't allow this to happen to you!

A much better answer should go something like this …

> **Interviewer:** I see that you observed doctors treating a case of dystonia. What was that like?
>
> **Candidate:** Dystonia was not a condition that I had come across before, but it was immediately clear that it was a high pressure situation that needed to be resolved immediately due to the nature of the condition. This particular case was severe, and the patient's neck had been twisted to the side. He was in a great deal of discomfort.
>
> **Interviewer:** What treatments are carried out for patients with these problems?

Candidate: In the emergency department, the patient was given a muscle relaxant to reduce the tension in the muscles and minimise the pain of the patient. This was not a recurrent situation for the patient and it was the first time he had experienced it, but the doctor was able to talk through the necessity for a referral to see a specialist neurologist. If the case can be put down to be an isolated incident, or not due to any particular disease, they might be treated with an injection of botulinum toxin directly into the affected muscles.

Interviewer: What is the botulinum toxin? Why would that be used?

Candidate: The botulinum toxin is produced by a type of bacteria known as Clostridium botulinum. The toxin blocks the release of the neurotransmitter acetylcholine at neuromuscular junctions. As a result, the muscle is unable to contract, which prevents dystonia.

Interviewer: What might the possible causative diseases be?

Candidate: My research has indicated that most commonly, the cause of dystonia remains unknown, though it is thought to be due to miscommunication between neurones in the brain. There are some neurodegenerative diseases, such as Parkinson's disease or multiple sclerosis, where dystonia is a symptom.

It can be difficult to persuade busy medical professionals to explain why they are carrying out each particular step. However, most will be willing to help, so time your questions accurately and approach members of the team who are most likely to provide you with the most insight.

Voluntary work

While work experience in a hospital or GP surgery is a useful way of identifying the key aspects of working as a doctor, it is also important to demonstrate your commitment to a career in medicine through more long-standing placements. Typically, these will be voluntary positions rather than work experience placements, and they will typically highlight the less glamorous aspects of a career in healthcare. A week spent helping elderly and confused patients walk to the toilet is worth a month in the hospital laboratory helping the technicians carry out routine tests.

Hospices and local care homes are usually happy to take on conscientious volunteers, and the work they do – caring for the terminally ill or the elderly – is particularly appropriate. Remember that you are not only working in these environments in order to learn about medicine in action. You are also there to prove, to yourself as well as to the admissions tutors, that you have the dedication and stomach for what is often an unpleasant and upsetting work environment. In completing work of this nature, you will be able to demonstrate your caring nature and develop your ability to deal with people.

> **TIP!**
>
> Because of health and safety regulations, it is not always possible to arrange work experience or voluntary work with GPs, in hospitals or in hospices. The medical schools' admissions tutors are aware of this but they will expect you to have found alternatives.

Voluntary work with a local charity is a good way of demonstrating your commitment as well as giving you the opportunity to find out more about medicine. The CEO of a leading charity confirmed this to us in a recent talk, when he said:

> 'The purpose of the voluntary sector is to help people in need. However, we need to help ourselves in order to survive as charities and continue to provide the support required by so many. Student volunteers are invaluable because they bring enthusiasm and purpose which the elderly respond to. While these work experiences are good for their applications to medical school, I would advise very strongly that they investigate the nature of the charity before they embark on it because work experience is only truly relevant and productive when you can connect to the work and the cause, not simply be undertaking it for the sake of ticking boxes.'

Contact details for some of the respective charities can be found at the end of this book, although the list is by no means exhaustive.

As with work experience, it is important to note down key experiences whilst undertaking voluntary work. You should be sure to ask any questions that you might have and jot down the answers that you are given. It is also worth making a note of the dates and durations of your placements, as this will show that you are actually committed to working in a caring role, rather than merely completing placements to tick a box on your application form.

How work experience and voluntary work support your application

When you come to write the personal statement section of your UCAS application, you will need to reflect on your practical experience of medicine. While you will need to communicate what you did or what you observed, it is important not to simply list things. The admissions tutors will be looking for what you were able to take away from the experience in terms of what you learned about yourself, key aspects of a doctor's daily life and any attributes that they exhibited that made them good at their job. It is likely that some medical schools will question you about the contents of your personal statement, so it is important that you are able to talk in more depth about the points you mention.

For example, if you were to write: 'During the year that I worked on Sunday evenings at St Sebastian's Hospice, I saw a number of patients who were suffering from cancer and it was interesting to observe the treatment they received and watch its effects.' A generous interviewer will ask you about the management of cancer, and you have an opportunity to impress if you can explain the use of drugs, radiotherapy, diet, exercise, etc. The other benefit of work in a medical environment is that you may be able to make a good impression on the senior staff you have worked for. If they are prepared to write a brief reference and send it to your school, the teacher writing your reference will be able to quote from it.

Work experience and voluntary work during the Coronavirus pandemic

As the Coronavirus pandemic continues to disrupt our daily lives, there is no doubt that it will also impact a student's ability to acquire work experience, especially in the field of medicine. Departments are limiting the number of non-frontline staff for safety reasons, making it even more difficult to gain access to these highly sought-after positions. While it's not an ideal scenario, most medical schools have recognised that getting a set amount of work experience could be problematic and have lifted any specific requirements. If you have found yourself in a situation where you have not been able to undertake a work experience placement in a medical setting, you should contact the admissions department to clarify that they will still consider your application, though they should be sympathetic given the gravity of the situation.

That being said, medical school admissions officers will still be looking for an in-depth understanding of the medical profession, including what the career entails and the values and skills required to be a doctor, so you will need to be creative in your approach to gaining this understanding. As well as talking to doctors and medical students, there are numerous online resources that will assist you in obtaining this knowledge. Free virtual medical work experience is now being provided by both Brighton and Sussex Medical School and the Royal College of General Practitioners. While they are not designed to replace face-to-face work experience entirely, completing these programmes could be vital in the current climate.

Virtual Work Experience Platform: Observe GP

Observe GP is a virtual learning experience for aspiring UK-based medics that provides an alternative to face-to-face work experience. The programme is organised by the Royal College of General Practitioners (RCGP) and supported by the Medical Schools Council. It is an interactive video platform that sets out to establish some of the realities of practising medicine as a GP, as well as the attributes required. It should take around 2.5 hours to complete, so it is worth looking into even if you have acquired face-to-face work experience!

More information can be found at www.rcgp.org.uk/training-exams/discover-general-practice/observe-gp.aspx.

Virtual Work Experience Platform: Brighton and Sussex Medical School

Brighton and Sussex Medical School recognised the importance of aspiring medical students gaining work experience, but also the limitations around accessing it for many people. As such, they set up their virtual work experience platform to give an insight into six medical specialities, including key attributes of the doctors and both the benefits and challenges of working within that speciality. The course should take up to 9 hours to complete.

More information can be found at https://bsmsoutreach.thinkific.com/courses/VWE.

Other things that you can do to support your application in the midst of a pandemic include the following.

- **Keep an eye on the news.** Throughout the pandemic, the media has covered many aspects of how it is affecting the NHS, from presenting facts and figures to giving an insight into how healthcare workers have been impacted. Some media sources will put a political spin on their stories, so you will need to see past this and read from a variety of sources to get a balanced view.
- **Voluntary work.** As with work experience, voluntary work within the NHS is likely to be disrupted, but the pandemic has brought about other voluntary opportunities that are certainly worth exploring. The purpose of voluntary work is to gain an insight into care work, as well as learning about your own skills and attributes. Providing it is safe for you to do so, you could explore whether any local community groups require support, or perhaps offer online opportunities, such as support groups. Nextdoor and Do-It.org are both organisations that coordinate voluntary work.

- **Independent learning.** Practising medicine involves a life-long commitment to learning, so taking it upon yourself to learn something medicine-related can demonstrate that you are willing to do this. This can involve reading around topics of interest online, such as through the *British Medical Journal*'s open access information, listening to podcasts or watching relevant TED Talks. You could also complete an online course, such as those provided by FutureLearn (www.futurelearn.com), which usually run over a period of a few weeks.

- **Online resources and social media.** Beyond the virtual work experience platforms detailed on page 35, many student and junior doctors present their journeys through social media platforms such as YouTube and Instagram, as well as through blogs. While these are more informal, they can still provide a useful insight into the realities of medicine as a career.

The Medical Schools Council have released guidance on gaining relevant experience for medicine applications during the time of Covid-19. This guide can be accessed at www.medschools.ac.uk/media/2717/a-guide-for-gaining-relevant-experience-during-the-pandemic.pdf.

They will also want to see that you understand the qualities required to succeed as a doctor, such as effective communication and being able to interact with a wide range of people. It would therefore be useful to consider the NHS Constitution, the details of which can be found here: www.gov.uk/government/publications/the-nhs-constitution-for-england.

3 | Deciding where to apply

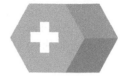

Prior to submitting your application to medical school, it is essential that you conduct careful research into the application process, entrance requirements, the nature of the work that you will be conducting as a doctor, and the skills and traits that you will be required to demonstrate. If you have a thorough understanding of each of these aspects, your decision to study medicine will be a well-informed one and, for the most part, should improve your chances of gaining a place.

Choosing a medical school

Once you have made the decision to study medicine, you will need to carefully research medical schools. There are various factors that might influence your decision.

- The way that the course is delivered (such as whether the course is integrated, traditional, CBL or PBL).
- The academic requirements (including GCSE and A level require-ments).
- The admissions tests that are required (either the UCAT or BMAT).
- The location of the university.
- The type of university.

You can obtain this information in a number of ways.

Online

A straightforward way of accessing information relating to the medical schools in the UK is using the UCAS website (www.ucas.com), which will often have links to the university websites too. It is important that you commit some time to exploring the information provided on both sites to find the information that you require. This information changes regularly, so if you are researching in advance, check back to make sure that nothing has changed closer to the time that you are submitting your application. If you are unable to get the answers you need from the internet, do not hesitate to contact the medical school either over the phone or via email.

An important point to note is that some medical schools offer more than one medicine course, including standard undergraduate degrees, post-graduate degrees and Foundation degrees. Make sure that you are looking at the appropriate course when conducting your research.

Open days

As well as researching medical schools online, you can also learn a great deal about them by visiting on open days. Information about open days can be obtained from university websites, or websites such as www.opendays.com. By attending an organised open day, you will be able to see the departments in which you will be studying and meet current academic staff and students, who will be able to answer any questions that you might have. You can also get a feel for the university in question – you will be spending the next five years of your life there, so it is important that you feel comfortable in that environment. If you don't, you might struggle to see the course through, irrespective of your academic achievements.

If you are planning on attending an open day, it is important that you ensure that you book onto any relevant talks to give yourself the best possible chance of obtaining the information that you need.

If you are unable to attend an organised open day, you should contact the university and ascertain whether there are any other opportunities to visit the department. In many cases, there will be someone who is able to meet you and give you a brief tour. If this is not possible, you can still visit on an informal basis to have a look around the university and see whether you like it, though you may not be able to visit the medical school itself.

Virtual Open Days

In light of the Coronavirus pandemic, many universities have converted their open days into virtual events that are conducted wholly online in order to protect the health of prospective students. A virtual open day is different to visiting a campus in person, yet still an excellent opportunity to see what a university has to offer and get an insight into a place where you might choose to study. While some universities will look to reinstate face-to-face open days in the coming months, virtual open days will persist and rightly so, as they have many benefits.

As you won't have to factor in travelling to the universities, you can attend more virtual open days than you might have initially intended, thus widening your options.

Virtual open days have differing formats depending on the university, but typically provide an opportunity to look at virtual tours, attend online webinars and talk to current students, lecturers and admissions officers, allowing you to ask any questions that you might have.

League tables

Another useful source of information regarding medical schools is university league tables, of which there are many available. The table below is compiled by the *Complete University Guide*, and bases its rankings on scores of student satisfaction, research quality and graduate prospects.

Table 2 Medical School rankings 2021

Medical school	Rank
University of Dundee	1
University of Glasgow	2
University of Oxford	3
University of Aberdeen	4
University of Edinburgh	5
Queen Mary, University of London	6
University of Cambridge	7
University of St Andrews	8
Imperial College London	9
Swansea University	10
University College London	11
University of Bristol	12
Newcastle University	13
Queen's University Belfast	14
Keele University	15
University of Exeter	16
University of Warwick	17
Cardiff University	18
Brighton and Sussex Medical School	19
University of Sheffield	20
Lancaster University	21
University of Birmingham	22
University of Leeds	23
University of Leicester	24
King's College London	25
University of Nottingham	26
University of Southampton	27
University of Plymouth	28
University of East Anglia	29
St George's, University of London	30
University of Manchester	31
University of Liverpool	32
Hull York Medical School	33
University of Buckingham	34
University of Central Lancashire	35

Source: www.thecompleteuniversityguide.co.uk/league-tables/rankings?s=medicine.
Reprinted with kind permission from the Complete University Guide.

NB: League tables do not give a full picture and should be viewed only as one element of the decision-making process, rather than using it solely. In addition, different league tables use different information to rank medical schools, so it is worth looking into what exactly the positioning is based on. In reality, there is no bad medical school – all of those that deliver medicine degrees are approved by the General Medical Council.

MSC-approved medical schools

There are currently 41 medical schools or university departments of medicine in the UK that are recognised by the Medical Schools Council (MSC). These medical schools are summarised in Table 11 (pages 221–224). The London School of Hygiene and Tropical Medicine is also recognised by the MSC, but is not discussed here, since it provides only postgraduate qualifications in specific areas of medicine. Of these universities, the majority are accredited by the General Medical Council (GMC), while there are several schools in the UK currently under review. These schools include:

- Anglia Ruskin School of Medicine
- Aston Medical School
- Brunel Medical School
- Edge Hill University Medical School
- Kent and Medway Medical School
- Scottish Graduate Entry to Medicine (ScotGEM), a combination of the University of St Andrews and the University of Dundee
- University of Sunderland School of Medicine.

For many of these medical schools, a number of restrictions applied to their first cohorts. For example, at Aston University, these places were limited to widening-participation students from the local area and international students for the first intake; as of 2019, Aston University will take applications from domestic students nationally. Anglia Ruskin University was also approved by the GMC for opening in 2018, and 100 students gained a place outside of the standard UCAS cycle in September of the same year. For 2021 entry, there will be places available for both domestic and international students at each of the new UK medical schools. However, it is always important to conduct research into any medical schools to which you are considering applying to ensure that there are no restrictions in place.

The University of Central Lancashire offers the majority of its places to international students, though a limited number of places are available to UK students resident in the north-west of England.

Brunel Medical School is newly established for 2021 entry, and will run a five-year undergraduate degree in medicine. In its first academic year, it will only be open to international students, but they intend to discuss places for UK students with Health Education England and the Office for Students imminently.

While these universities are not yet accredited by the GMC, they are approved. Put simply, this means that the degrees obtained from these universities are not yet recognised for the practice of medicine in the UK, but this is standard for new medical schools; they do not become accredited until the first cohort has graduated. However, the GMC closely regulates the delivery of these degrees and annual reviews are available on the GMC website. You should not be put off by the lack of GMC accreditation of a medicine programme; in fact, each of the medical schools discussed above is guaranteed by an established medical school, meaning that if anything were to go wrong, you would graduate from the guarantor medical school instead.

The University of Buckingham, a privately funded university, is recognised by the MSC. It was added to the GMC's accredited list of universities in May 2019 following the graduation of its first cohort of students. Swansea University and Warwick Medical School also appear on the MSC list, although they only offer Graduate Entry (A101) programmes.

The universities on the list offer a range of options for students wishing to study medicine:

- five- or six-year MBBS or MBChB courses (UCAS codes A100 or A106)
- four-year accelerated graduate-entry courses (A101, A102 or A109)
- six-year courses that include a 'pre-med' year (A103 or A104).

Entry requirements of all medical schools are also summarised in Table 11 (pages 221–224).

New medical school places

The number of recognised medical schools in the UK increased in 2018 due to a government initiative to increase the number of medical school places available to students by 25%, demonstrating that the NHS will have the necessary provisions in place as it continues to expand in the coming years. Some 1,500 additional places were allocated to both existing medical schools and five new medical schools.

The five new medical schools were:

- The University of Sunderland
- Edge Hill University
- Anglia Ruskin University
- University of Lincoln
- Canterbury Christ Church University and University of Kent.

The impact of Covid-19 on medical school places

Results day in August 2020 was an unpleasant time for many aspiring medics. Students in this cohort were unable to sit their exams following their cancellation, and English studemts were instead awarded calculated grades based on an Ofqual-derived algorithm. Many of these students found themselves with much lower grades than they had anticipated which led to them losing their hard-earned medical school places. As with any other year, medical schools were then tasked with filling places in the days following results day. Despite promising that there would be no U-turn on results, the Government ultimately decided that they would instead award the highest grade out of the calculated grade, Centre Assessed Grade (CAG) – the grade the school submitted for them – and the grade achieved in an October resit exam. With CAGs being awarded, there were many more students who had met the conditions of their offers than places available. As such, this meant that many students who had met the conditions of their offer were not guaranteed a place for 2020 entry.

To assist with the placement of successful students, the Department for Education agreed to lift the cap on medical school places and provided confirmation of additional funding to support both university and clinical placements. While this was a positive move, it left many questions regarding placements for 2021, as successful candidates had their places deferred and the 2021 applicant cohort have had their A level studies significantly disrupted by Covid-19, with 2021 examinations cancelled. Despite the increased intake for 2020 and a number of places being deferred for 2021, medical schools intend to recruit in line with their normal numbers for 2021 entry at the time of writing, with pressure on the Department for Education to provide additional places for a second year in a row.

Factors to consider when choosing a medical school

You can apply to up to four medical schools in one application cycle. In deciding which ones to eliminate, you may find the following points helpful.

- **Grades and retakes.** If you are worried that you will not achieve a minimum of three A grades at A level the first time round, it is worth doing some careful research into which universities consider retake candidates (see Table 11, pages 221–224). While there is an increasing number of medical schools that will consider students who are retaking their A levels, some will only consider your application a second time if you applied to them in the first instance, or if you secured particular grades the first time around.

- **Interviews.** All medical schools interview A level candidates; some still use traditional panel interviews, while the majority use Multiple Mini Interviews (MMIs). Each school's interview policy is shown in Table 12 (see pages 225–227).
- **Location and socialising.** You may be attracted to the idea of being at a campus university rather than at one of the medical schools that are not located on the campuses of their affiliated universities. One reason for this may be that you would like to mix with students from a wide variety of disciplines and that you will enjoy the intellectual and social cross-fertilisation. However, it is worth keeping in mind that medical school hours and demands are arduous, so identifying a university solely based on opportunities for socialising is not advised!
- **Course structure.** While all the medical schools are well equipped and provide a high standard of teaching, there are real differences in the way the courses are taught and examined and you will not find two the same. Specifically, the majority offer an integrated course in which students see patients at an early stage and certainly before the formal clinical part of the course. The other main distinction is between systems-based courses (e.g. Manchester and Liverpool), which teach medicine in terms of the body's systems (e.g. the cardiovascular system), and subject-based courses (e.g. Oxford and Cambridge), which teach in terms of the fundamental subjects (anatomy, biochemistry, etc.).
- **Teaching style.** The style of teaching can also vary from place to place. See pages 10–22 for more information on PBL, CBL, integrated and traditional approaches to teaching.
- **Intercalated degrees and electives.** Another difference in the courses offered concerns the opportunities for an intercalated Honours degree and electives. The Intercalated degree scheme allows students to tack on one further year of study either to the end of the two-year pre-clinical course or as an integrated part of a six-year course. Successful completion of this year, which may be used to study a wide variety of subjects, confers an Honours degree qualification. Electives are periods of work experience away from the medical school and, in some cases, abroad. See pages 22–25 for more information.

Academic requirements

By the time you read this you will probably have chosen your GCSE subjects or even taken them. If not, here are some points to consider.

- While there are obviously exceptions, most universities specify particular grades (typically A/7 or B/6) in English language, maths and science subjects (whether dual, triple or core and additional). You will need to carefully research the requirements for each medical school and ensure that you meet the requirements before applying there. Many medical schools ask for a 'good' set of GCSE results. What this means exactly varies considerably from university to university, but on average, a minimum of five GCSEs at grade A/7 or B/6, including the aforementioned core subjects.

- Most medical schools require the study of chemistry, plus at least one other science (biology or physics) or maths. For the most part, the second science subject requested is usually biology. However, there is an increasing amount of flexibility with subject choices, with a number of universities no longer stating chemistry as an A level requirement. At the time of writing, these universities include Anglia Ruskin, East Anglia, Keele, Kent, Lancaster, Leeds, Leicester, Manchester, Newcastle, Plymouth, Queen Mary, Sheffield, South- ampton and Sunderland, though it is important to closely check university websites at the time.

- If AS level examinations are completed, these are likely to be taken into account by the admissions tutors reviewing your application. If it is your school's policy to sit these exams in year 12, it is important to remember that they are stand-alone qualifications and should therefore be taken seriously.

If you have already taken your GCSEs and achieved disappointing grades, you should carefully research the requirements of each univer- sity at GCSE level and identify the universities where you have the best possible chance. If it is genuinely the case, your referee can vouch for you and indicate in your reference that your A level attainment is unlikely to be a reflection of your GCSE performance. To do so, it is crucial that you work extremely hard to prove that this is the case as soon as your A levels begin.

In the case of mitigating circumstances that have impacted your attain- ment at GCSE, you should contact the university admissions department to ascertain what the required procedure is in that situation. For the most part, a comment from your teacher in your reference will be suffi- cient, but they may also require a separate form or letter including evidence of the circumstances before they will consider your application.

AS levels

Given that the policy for most schools is that AS level examinations are not compulsory, the general stance for medical schools is that AS grades will no longer be part of any offers made and they do not have an explicit AS grade requirement. However, Queen's University Belfast will judge a candidate's application on whether they have been able to sit a fourth AS exam at their school.

If AS levels are included in the application, they will serve as a reason- able indicator of anticipated attainment overall, so it is likely that admissions tutors may consider them if they are present on the application. As such, it is crucially important that you work hard from the start of the course so that you are thoroughly prepared for AS examinations, as they will form a part of your application, even though they do not contribute to your overall A level grade.

A level choices

Your choice of A levels

You will see from Table 11 (pages 221–224) that all medical schools now ask for just two science/maths subjects at A level, with the majority still requiring biology and chemistry. When choosing your A level subjects, there are three important considerations.

1. Choose subjects that you are good at. You must be capable of an A grade as a minimum requirement. If you aren't sure, ask your teachers.
2. Choose subjects that will help you in your medical course; life at medical school is tough enough as it is without having to learn new subjects from scratch.
3. It is wholly acceptable to choose a non-scientific third subject that you enjoy and that will provide you with an interesting topic of conversation at your interview. With the exception of general studies, critical thinking and, in many cases, further maths, universities do not discriminate based on the third subject. Students who can cope with the differing demands of arts and sciences at A level have an advantage in that they can demonstrate breadth.

So what combination of subjects should you choose? In addition to chemistry/biology and another science at A level, you might also consider subjects such as psychology, sociology or a language. In the reforms, psychology as a subject became more mathematical, as well as scientific; as such, Edge Hill University, Keele University, the Kent and Medway Medical School, Lancaster University, the University of Leicester, the University of Manchester, Plymouth University and the University of Sheffield will now regard it as a second science subject in their grade offers. The point to bear in mind when you are making your choices is that you need high grades, so do not pick a subject that sounds interesting, such as Italian, if you are not good at languages. Similarly, although an A level in further maths might look good on your UCAS application, you will need to consider if it is actually something universities want you to have. You will need to check the individual requirements; most medical schools will indicate preferred A level subjects in addition to science A levels.

Taking four A levels

There's no harm in doing more than three A levels (and an AS exam, if offered by your school), but there is really no advantage to it. In most cases, the added pressure of studying for a fourth A level means that you run the risk of pulling down your overall grade, so you might consider dropping the additional qualification at the end of year 12. Medical schools will not include the fourth A level in any conditional offers they make.

If you are taking the International Baccalaureate, then you should still be aiming to take biology and chemistry, as these are the subjects required for undergraduate study. However, some universities specify chemistry and one of maths, biology, human biology and physics. If you are not taking these subjects, you should be considering what makes you think you will be able to cope on a medicine course. For Scottish students, you are expected to have at least two Advanced Highers and three Highers, with biology and chemistry and usually either maths or physics as well to at least Higher level; Imperial College, for example, asks for five Highers and three Advanced Highers to A grade standard. Overall, students should be aiming for majority A grades in Highers and Advanced Highers, though AB at Advanced Highers is accepted, or even BB in the case of the University of Edinburgh, for example.

The prediction

The admissions tutor will look for a grade prediction in the reference that your teacher writes about you. Your teacher will make a prediction based on the reports of your subject teachers, your GCSE grades and, most importantly, the results of any exams taken at the end of year 12.

Consequently, it is vital that you work hard during the first year of A levels. Only by doing so will you get the reference you need. If there is any reason or excuse to explain why you did badly at GCSE or did not work hard in year 12, you must make sure that the teacher writing your reference knows about it and includes it in the reference. The most common reasons for poor performance are illness and problems at home (e.g. illness of a close relation or family breakdown). In many cases, additional evidence will be required by the university to support this claim, so stating that you underperformed due to ill health when this is not the case is likely to cause bigger problems.

The bottom line is that you need to persuade your school that you are on track for grades of AAA or higher, depending on where you are applying. Convincing everyone else usually involves convincing yourself!

Non-medical choices

Although you can apply to a total of five institutions through UCAS, you may apply to only four medical schools. What should you do with the final slot? Applying for an alternative, non-medical course will not jeopardise your medicine application in any way, but the fifth choice is still worthy of careful consideration for a number of reasons. There are two main options regarding the fifth choice.

1. Do not include a fifth choice

If you are truly committed to becoming a doctor, you need to consider whether you would realistically accept whichever course you include as a fifth choice. If you know that you would not consider that course in place of medicine and would prefer to reapply, it may be in your best interests to leave the final choice blank. If you were then unfortunate enough to not secure a place to study medicine, you could spend a year developing your application in order to boost your chances the following academic year.

2. Carefully consider an alternative course

You might choose to include a non-medical choice on your form if you are not prepared to wait for a year if your application is unsuccessful, or if you intend to enter medicine as a graduate (see below).

Trying to combine two different subjects in your personal statements is a recipe for disaster. While admissions tutors cannot see which other courses you have applied for on your UCAS application, it will automatically signal to both departments that you are not really committed to either course. This would be especially apparent if you were including a subject such as chemical engineering or archaeology as your fifth choice. As such, under no circumstances should this be done; simply stick to medicine with the personal statement in your UCAS application.

If there is a course that you would genuinely consider studying in place of medicine, or perhaps you are already reapplying and just want to go to university next academic year, there are ways of applying to two separate courses. For the most part, students will want to apply to another science-based course, which minimises the problems associated with the personal statement. However, it does not completely eradicate them.

If you do intend to include a fifth choice which you would genuinely consider in the case of an unsuccessful medicine application, then you may need to contact the university in question to ascertain whether or not they will consider this application. Many universities will happily consider this option once you have contacted them to explain why your personal statement does not match up with the course, but some may request an additional personal statement. In this case, you must be prepared to deliver a second personal statement outlining why you are committed to studying that course if you are to successfully acquire a place. This is becoming especially common where students choose other vocational degrees, such as pharmacy or optometry, as their back-up choices.

Many students now pursue the option of undertaking a first degree in a related subject, such as biomedical science, which they then utilise as a platform to gain access onto medicine as a second degree.

To BSc ... or not to BSc?

As discussed above, many students who are initially unsuccessful in their pursuit of medicine will undertake a related science degree first, such as biomedical science or biochemistry. Whether or not to consider a BSc in lieu of a medicine degree is a very tricky question, but ultimately, it can be answered by no one other than you. There are several pros and cons worth considering.

Cons

- You might spend a whole three years on a course you never really wanted to study. Studying a subject at degree level is an enormous commitment, and if you are not entirely motivated by the content, it can be a very trying time.
- Three years of study will add additional cost and time before actually getting into medical school.
- Entry to medical school after graduating is not guaranteed.
- If admitted to undergraduate medical school only, you will still have to study for five more years.
- You might lose focus on medicine if you study something else first.
- You may not get the student funding and help towards fees, compared with if you go straight after A levels.

Pros

- Many BSc degrees are in biomedical or medical school – if you don't enjoy this, would you enjoy medicine, which is not that different? There are also two-year BSc courses designed for medicine.
- Medicine is a life-long commitment, so two to three years of additional study should not worry you. Becoming a good doctor is a journey, not a target.
- Although entry to medical school is not guaranteed, some BSc courses do offer a very secure pathway to overseas medical schools in the event you don't get into the UK.
- Applying as a graduate certainly makes your medical school application stronger as you have matured as an individual and academically.
- Having a BSc as well as a medical degree may enhance your chances to get the medical job you desire – a reason why many medical students intercalate.
- Studying a first degree will give you time to mature as a person. You will become acquainted with the demands of university life and develop your skills in independent study. Many students who take this approach find that by the time they reach medical school, they are more comfortable with the workload and can approach the study of medicine with greater confidence.

Applying to Oxbridge medical schools

Oxbridge is in a separate category because, if getting into most medical schools is difficult, entry into Oxford or Cambridge is even more so (the extra hurdles facing students wishing to apply to Oxford or Cambridge are discussed in *Getting into Oxford & Cambridge*, another guide in this series). The general advice given here also applies to Oxbridge, but the competition is intense, and before you include either university on your UCAS application you need to be confident that you can achieve the entrance standard grades (A*A*A at Cambridge and A*AA at Oxford) at A level and that you will interview well.

You cannot apply to both Oxford and Cambridge in your application and your teachers will advise you whether to apply to either. You should discuss an application to Oxford or Cambridge with your teachers at an early stage. You would need a good reason to apply to Oxbridge against the advice of your teachers and it certainly is not worth applying on the 'off chance' of getting in. By doing so you will simply waste one of your valuable four choices.

When considering an Oxbridge application, you must carefully consider which of the two universities you will apply to, and in addition, the college at which you are interested in studying. There is no disadvantage to submitting an open application, which means that each college can consider your application and invite you to interview. An important distinction between Oxford and Cambridge and other universities is their tutorial system. You will meet with a tutor, alongside two or three other medicine students from your college, to discuss a particular topic in great depth. These sessions are often accompanied by a significant amount of work specific to each college.

Both Oxford and Cambridge will be looking for all of the attributes in your application that show that you will make an outstanding doctor. It is also worth remembering, however, that the elite universities are highly academic, so it may be worth adding in a little extra in your applications. This may be associated with areas of research that interest you, or wider reading that you have conducted in specific areas of medicine.

4 | The UCAS application

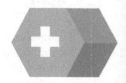

There are various components to a medicine application that will ultimately determine whether or not you are made an offer. The first component of the application to study medicine in the UK is completion of the UCAS application form. Some sections of the application are purely factual, such as your name, address and prior examination results, as well as a section where you enter your choice of medical schools. Perhaps most importantly, you must include a personal statement, which gives you an opportunity to write about why you want to study medicine and what would make you a good fit for the course and career. In addition, a teacher will provide a reference which supports your application.

The application is critical, as this is what the admissions tutors at each university that you apply to will receive. On reviewing your application, the admissions tutors will make a decision as to whether or not you will be invited to interview. With the exception of one UK medical school, you will need to attend a face-to-face interview in order to gain a conditional offer.

What happens to your application

By the 15 October deadline, medical schools will have received an extremely high number of applications which far exceeds the number of places that they have. Some UK medical schools can receive up to almost ten times as many applications as they have places, which admissions tutors will then review to ascertain who deserves the opportunity to prove themselves at interview. Admissions tutors have the ruthless task of culling applications that are insufficient, and painstakingly reviewing those that remain.

Most medical schools have a well-defined set of criteria which students should consider before submitting an application. Typically, the first part of the selection process by admissions tutors will be ruling out any applicant who does not meet these criteria in full, so it is crucial that you take the time to check that this is the case. The majority of admissions tutors are happy to discuss these aspects of the application with you, so make sure that you conduct your research in good time and where necessary, get in touch with them to see whether you are eligible.

For the most part, students applying to medicine will have been pre-dicted the required grades (which are typically AAA or higher), or in some circumstances, may have obtained them already. In addition, a high proportion of applicants will have a good set of GCSE or equivalent results. The academic demands are consistently high with medicine, so it is unlikely that academic attainment alone will be sufficient to make your application stand out.

This is where the rest of your application comes in, and in particular, your personal statement and academic reference. The personal state-ment should discuss your motivation to study medicine, as well as your work experience or voluntary work and what undertaking it has taught you about working in this particular healthcare setting. Your reference, usually provided by a teacher at your school, will then discuss your strengths as a student.

In order to decide who to call for interview, the admissions tutors will have to make a decision based solely on the information presented to them. If your application does not demonstrate the necessary require-ments at this stage, irrespective of how outstanding your personal qualities are, you will not be invited to interview, which means that the university in question cannot make you an offer. Historically, the University of Edinburgh has not based its decisions on face-to-face interviews, however the university announced that for 2020 entry it would be introducing a face-to-face selection process in the form of an assessment day.

The sample medical interview selection form on page 53 gives an example of the ways in which your application might be viewed by admissions tutors. When preparing to apply, it might be worth you using this as a rough way of assessing your own application, and identifying ways in which you could strengthen it.

UCAS Apply

When you apply for UK universities, you do so using the UCAS Apply system. The online UCAS form is accessed through the UCAS website (www.ucas.com). You register online either through your school or college, or as a private individual. Some of the information that you provide on the form is factual, such as where you live, where you have studied, what academic qualifications you have, details of examinations that you are going to take, and which university courses you are apply-ing for. Other sections, such as the personal statement and reference, allow more expansive information to be communicated. The sections of the UCAS form are as follows.

- Personal Details: this includes all of your basic personal information as well as contact details and details of criminal convictions and any special educational needs.

- Additional Information: in this section, you enter details of your ethnicity, parental occupations and details of any activities that you have completed in preparation for higher education.
- Student Finance: this section asks about your intention to apply for student finance and if you wish your details to be shared automatically with loan providers.
- Choices: this is where you enter your course choices.
- Education: this section is used to provide details of all of the schools and colleges you have attended (not including primary school) and the details of the qualifications you have received there.
- Employment: in this section, include details of any paid employment.
- Personal Statement: finally, this is where you put your personal statement once it is completed.
- Reference and Predicted Grades: this is where your academic referee enters their reference about you and the grades you have been predicted for each subject.

Once your form is complete, it is accessed by the person who will write your reference; they then check it, add the reference and predicted grades and send it to UCAS. Remember, that when you have completed your form and press 'send', the form does not go straight to UCAS, but is instead sent to the person who oversees the UCAS process at your school. This means that your form can get returned to you at this point if there are any mistakes that need correcting.

Despite the help that the electronic version provides, it is still possible to create an unfavourable impression on the admissions tutors through spelling mistakes, grammatical errors and unclear personal statements. In order to ensure that this does not happen, follow these tips.

- Read the instructions for each section of the application carefully before filling it in.
- Double-check all dates (when you joined and left schools, when you sat examinations), examination boards, GCSE grades and personal details (fee codes, residential status codes, disability codes).
- Plan your personal statement as you would an essay. Lay it out in a logical order. Make the sentences short and to the point. Split the section into paragraphs, covering each of the necessary topics (i.e. reasons for wanting to study medicine, work experience and voluntary work, academic interests and extracurricular activities and achievements). This will enable the selectors to read and assess it quickly and easily.
- Ask your teachers to cast a critical eye over your draft, and don't be too proud to make changes in the light of their advice.

Once your application has been submitted, you can keep track of the responses from the universities using UCAS Track.

MEDICAL INTERVIEW SELECTION FORM
Name: UCAS number: Age at entry: Gap year?: Selector: Date:

SELECTION CRITERIA COMMENTS
1 Academic (score out of 10) GCSE results/AS grades/A level predictions UCAT/BMAT result 2 Commitment (score out of 10) Genuine interest in medicine? Relevant work experience? Community involvement? 3 Personal (score out of 10) Range of interests? Involvement in school activities? Achievements and/or leadership? Referee supports application?
Total score (maximum of 30):

Recommendation of selector:	Interview	Score 25–30
	Reserve list	Score 16–24
	Rejection	Score 0–15

Further comments (if any):

Figure 3 Sample candidate selection form

Timing

The main UCAS submission period is from 8 September to 15 January, but medical applications have to be with UCAS by 15 October. Late applications are also permitted, although medical schools are not bound to consider them. Remember that most referees take at least a week to consult the relevant teachers and compile a reference, so allow for that and aim to submit your application by mid-September unless there is a good reason for delaying.

The only convincing reason for delaying is that your teachers cannot predict high A level grades at the moment, but might be able to do so if they see high-quality work during the autumn term. If you are not being predicted the minimum grades required, it does not necessarily mean that you won't be able to apply, but it will require some careful research and contact with admissions tutors to establish whether or not you would be considered.

Interviews usually take place between November and March of the academic year and so if you have not heard by January, it is not necessarily a negative situation.

The reference

The reference will be written by a referee who could be your headteacher, housemaster, personal tutor or head of sixth form. They will write about what an outstanding person you are and about your contribution to school life as well as your academic achievement (i.e. on target for at least three A grades at A level), and they will then also give reasons why you are suitable to study medicine. For them to say this it must of course be true, as referees have to be as honest as possible and they will accurately assess your character and potential to succeed at university. You must have demonstrated to your teachers and other members of staff that you have all the necessary qualities required to become a doctor.

Ideally, your efforts to impress them will have begun at the start of the sixth form (or preferably before this); you will have become involved in school activities, while at the same time working hard on your A level subjects and developing strong interpersonal skills, demonstrated by your interactions with staff and students. If you do not feel as though you have done this, don't worry, because it is never too late. Some people mature later than others, so if this does not sound like you, start to make efforts to get involved in the wider life of your school or college, as this will help provide evidence for the people who will contribute to your reference.

To what extent does your referee support your application?

It is vitally importance to express your utmost gratitude to your referee and make sure that they know all the good news about your work in hospitals and in the local community. Remember that the teacher writing your reference will rely heavily on advice from other teachers too. You can help yourself by working hard, looking keen and talking about medicine, where relevant, in class. Ask questions that display your genuine interest in becoming a doctor or a particular topic, as well as thinking beyond the confines of the syllabus in class and ask intelligent, medicine-related questions such as those given below. Do not try and ask complicated medical questions for the sake of it; ask questions because you genuinely wish to know the answer and could carry on the conversation once given the answer.

- How effective is gene therapy in the treatment of cystic fibrosis?
- How does being obese actually contribute to suffering from type II diabetes?
- Is it because enzymes become denatured at over 45°C that patients suffering from heatstroke have to be cooled down quickly using ice?
- Could sex-linked diseases such as muscular dystrophy be avoided by screening the sperm to eliminate those containing the X chromosomes that carry the harmful recessive genes from an affected male?

If your referee is approachable, you should be able to ask whether they feel able to support your application. In the unlikely case that they cannot recommend you, you should consider asking if another teacher could complete the reference; clashes of personality do very occasionally occur and you must not let the medical schools receive a reference that damns you.

As part of the reference your referee will need to predict the grades that you are likely to achieve. The entry requirements of the medical schools are shown in Table 11 (pages 221–224). If you are predicted lower than the requirements it is almost certain that you will not be considered. Talk to your teachers and find out whether you are on target for these grades. If not, you may need to work harder to show them what you're capable of, or you may want to hold back on your application until you have achieved your grades.

If you are a mature student or going through graduate entry, the referee could be a lecturer from your university who will provide the appropriate information.

What happens next and what to do about it

Once your reference has been submitted, a receipt will be sent to your school or college to acknowledge its arrival. Your application is then processed and UCAS will send you confirmation of your details. If you don't receive this, you should check with your referee that it has been correctly submitted. The confirmation will contain your application number, your details and the list of courses to which you have applied.

Check carefully to make sure that the details in your application have been saved to the UCAS system correctly. At the same time, make a note of your UCAS number – you will need to quote this when you contact the medical schools.

Now comes a period of waiting, which can be very unsettling but which must not distract you from your studies. Most medical schools decide whether or not they want to interview you within a few months.

- If one or more of the medical schools decides to interview you, your next letter will be an invitation to visit the school and attend an interview. (For advice on how to prepare for the interview, see Chapter 6.)
- If you are unlucky, the next correspondence you get from UCAS will contain the news that you have been rejected by one or more of your chosen schools. Does a rejection mean it's time to relax on the A level work and dust off alternative plans? Should you be reading up on exactly what the four-year course in road resurfacing involves? No, you should not!

A rejection is a setback and it does make the path into medicine that bit steeper, but it isn't an excuse to give up. A rejection should act as a spur to work even harder because the grades you achieve at A level are now even more important. Don't give up and do turn to Chapter 8 to see what to do when you get your A level results.

Deferral of place

If you are going to apply to study medicine, you should expect to start as soon as possible, unless, and this is important, there is a good reason for you to make a deferral request. Bear in mind, universities are under no pressure to defer places as they put greater emphasis on places available for first-time applicants, except in extenuating circumstances. However, they do have roughly a 10% quota of students annually who will defer their places and they are sometimes happy to grant these requests if the student can prove they will be doing something worthwhile with their gap year. If there is a compelling reason, talk it through with them first to discuss your options there, as they will expect you to be undertaking something worthwhile in the intervening time.

Case study

Anushka is a fourth-year medical student at Lancaster University.

'My curiosity of the functioning of the human body, coupled with the rapidly evolving nature of medicine initiated my interest in becoming a doctor. Illnesses that were thought to be incurable are now being cured due to new discoveries being made. It is this that motivated me to pursue a career in medicine.

'Before applying to study medicine, I volunteered at my local care home and the British Heart Foundation charity shop. My main role at the care home was to help feed the residents, however I tried to be as involved as possible in all care needs of the residents. Work experience built my confidence and enhanced my communication skills. These key skills form the foundations of a doctor, and is something you can build as you progress in your career. In my opinion, the earlier you get exposure and experience in these skills, the better.

'Unfortunately, I did not achieve my A level grades that were required for entrance into medical school first time around. Enrolling at MPW was the best decision I have ever made. With their expertise and support, I was able to achieve my predicted grades in Biology, Chemistry and Mathematics of A*AA and get offers from two medical schools.

'I am thoroughly enjoying my time at medical school. Although it can be challenging at times, due to the vast quantity of work, once you establish your studying technique, you begin to appreciate your theoretical knowledge and clinical practice. It is rewarding to see conditions you have studied be treated when you attend placement in hospital.

'My medical school incorporates professional ethics into the medical course. I really enjoy this aspect as we have ethical case debates every year, in which doctors and students can participate.

'Medicine is an extensive subject, where it is impossible to know everything, yet difficult to ascertain how much depth is enough for your level. This can sometimes get quite overwhelming, and you may find yourself with little flexibility in your work–life balance.

'The pandemic has been an uncertain time for all of us. Due to the disruption of Covid-19, I have witnessed the flexibility of the NHS and how services have adapted to the changing times. It has provided me with the opportunity to gain invaluable experience in terms of learning about the care of patients with Covid-19 and its complications.

'Although I am unsure of the particular speciality I want to pursue in my career, within 10 years I would want to be in my speciality training, and potentially close to becoming a consultant.

'My top three tips for prospective medical students would be:

- Get work experience as early as possible in care homes, charity shops, GPs, etc.
- Make sure that you thoroughly prepare for interviews, with mock interviews at your school if possible.
- Do plenty of practice for your UCAT and BMAT entrance exams.'

Aptitude tests

Almost all UK medical schools ask applicants to sit aptitude tests as part of the application process. At undergraduate level, these tests include either the UCAT or the BMAT tests.

UCAT (University Clinical Aptitude Test)

From 2019, the test formerly known as UKCAT (UK Clinical Aptitude Test) has changed its name to the UCAT. The change affects the name alone, and has not influenced the timings or structure of the test itself.

The UCAT has been adopted by 30 universities as part of their admissions procedures, and helps them make an informed choice between the highest-performing candidates for undergraduate medical study. It is designed to ensure that students have the mental capabilities, attitude and professional conduct required for a career in the medical field. It is not a test of your curriculum knowledge or any scientific background. The UCAT tests thought processes and as such cannot be revised for, though it is possible to prepare yourself in order to boost your overall attainment.

The UCAT is a computer-based test , and this aspect of the test should not be underestimated: your eyes will get very tired after staring at a computer screen for two hours. So make sure that at least some of your preparation is done online.

The UCAT can be completed at an official Pearson VUE test centre or at home (UCAT Online) using Pearson VUE's online proctoring service. Careful consideration should be given as to where you sit the test. Sitting the test at home was brought in to ensure that the UCAT was still accessible to all students, despite the ongoing challenges that the Covid-19 pandemic presents.

If completing your test at a centre, the setting will be unfamiliar, but it provides a more formal testing environment that may reduce distractions and aid concentration, and it removes the possibility of technical failure. Test centres can be found in many locations worldwide, so it is worthwhile identifying which test centres are local and therefore convenient to you. If there is a problem with your attending any of these centres, you should consult the UCAT website (www.ucat.ac.uk).

Sitting the test at home gives greater flexibility in terms of choosing a test date, and it would eliminate the stress of travelling to an unfamiliar test centre. You may be more comfortable sitting your test at home, but you should consider possible distractions, whether your internet connection is sufficient and whether your device meets the technical requirements (this can be assessed using UCAT's System Test in advance). There are also a number of ID requirements that must be met to sit the UCAT Online, including identity and workspace verification and live proctoring, which involves using a webcam and microphone. If you are below the age of 18, a parent or guardian must be present when you begin your test.

Registration is typically open between May and September and in previous years it was possible to sit the test between early July and early October, though the earlier you take it, the better. By reserving an early slot, you will be able to sit the UCAT with a clear head, and it will give you more time to research which universities will consider your overall application, inclusive of the UCAT score. In addition, if you become unwell or are unable to make your booked test for any reason, you have the opportunity to reschedule for a later date. If you book your initial test too late in the cycle, then it is unlikely that there will be local slots remaining for you to complete it, meaning that you have to sit the test when you're ill or travel a considerable distance to take it!

Because of the Covid-19 pandemic, there was a shift in registration and testing dates in 2020, with registration opening at the beginning of July and testing starting at the beginning of August and finishing at the beginning of October. Applicants were encouraged to sit the UCAT early due to the pandemic and the uncertainty surrounding the testing situation should the UK find itself in a position of heightened cases with the potential for further lockdowns.

If you have any disabilities or additional needs that require you to have extra time in examinations, it is important that you register for the UCATSEN instead of the regular test. For example, if you require 25% additional time in examinations due to a diagnosis of dyslexia, the UCATSEN will allocate this additional time to each section of the exam. If you require special access arrangements for examinations, then you should directly contact Pearson VUE customer services to discuss these arrangements before you book the test.

There are five separately timed sections to the UCAT. These sections are based on a set of skills that medical (and dental) schools believe are vital to be successful as a medical practitioner.

1. **Verbal Reasoning.** Candidates are provided with a piece of text that they have to analyse and answer questions on. This section assesses the ability of the candidate to critically evaluate written information.
2. **Decision Making.** This test assesses a candidate's ability to apply logic to reach a decision or conclusion, evaluate arguments and analyse statistical information.
3. **Quantitative Reasoning.** This section assesses a candidate's ability to critically evaluate information presented in a numerical form.
4. **Abstract Reasoning.** Candidates are presented with a series of shapes that they must interpret and identify patterns within. This

section assesses the use of convergent and divergent thinking to infer relationships.

5. **Situational Judgement.** This tests candidates' ability to comprehend real-world situations and to identify critical factors and appropriate behaviour in handling them.

The test lasts two hours in total. Those candidates with special educational needs take the UCATSEN and are given the allocated additional time per section.

Table 3 Timings for UCAT/UCATSEN

Section	Items	Standard Test Time	Extra Time/ UCATSEN
Verbal Reasoning	44 items	22 minutes	27.5 minutes
Decision Making	29 items	32 minutes	40 minutes
Quantitative Reasoning	36 items	25 minutes	31.25 minutes
Abstract Reasoning	55 items	14 minutes	17.25 minutes
Situational Judgement	690 items	27 minutes	33.75 minutes
Total time		120 minutes	150 minutes

Dates

A list of important dates regarding the UCAT exam can be found at www.ucat.ac.uk. For those students wishing to apply for entry in 2022:

- registration opens: 2 June 2021
- test booking begins: 28 June 2021
- testing begins: 26 July 2021
- registration closes: 22 September 2021
- last testing date: 29 September 2021

Please note that these dates are subject to change. Please check the UCAT website for updates.

Universities that require the UCAT
Table 4 (opposite) shows the UK universities that require students to sit the UCAT as part of their application process.

Preparation
Although the UCAT website tries to discourage students from doing any preparation for the test other than sitting the practice tests available online, students who have sat the test in the past have found that the more practice they had on timed IQ-type tests, the better prepared they felt. In this chapter you will find practice questions for each section.

Table 4 Medical schools requiring UCAT admissions test

Medical school	UCAS course code
University of Aberdeen	A100, A105
Anglia Ruskin University	A100
University of Birmingham	A100, A101
University of Bristol	A100, A108
Cardiff University	A100, A104
University of Dundee	A100, A104
University of East Anglia	A100, A104
Edge Hill University	A100, A110
University of Edinburgh	A100
University of Exeter	A100
University of Glasgow	A100
Hull York Medical School	A100, A101
Keele University	A100, A104
Kent and Medway Medical School	A100
King's College London	A100, A101, A102
University of Leicester	A100, A199
University of Liverpool	A100
University of Manchester	A104, A106
Newcastle University	A100, A101
University of Nottingham	A100, A108
University of Plymouth (Peninsula Schools of Medicine and Dentistry)	A100
Queen Mary University of London	A100, A101, A110, A120
Queen's University Belfast	A100
University of Sheffield	A100, A101
University of Southampton	A100, A101, A102
University of St Andrews	A100, A990
St George's, University of London	A100
University of Sunderland	A100
University of Warwick	A101

General hints

- Use the practice questions provided on the following pages to familiarise yourself with the type of questions that are asked and the time constraints in the test. It is important to practise the different types of question available so that you can improve your approach to each question type.
- Most candidates have great difficulty completing the sections of the test in the allocated time, so don't panic if you find that this is the case when you are practising questions. The UCAT website provides practice tests that can be completed online, and these give a realistic representation of the level of questioning you will get in the

official exam, as well as the timing and the practical aspects of completing tests on a computer.

- There is a point for each right answer, but no points are deducted for wrong answers.

- Try not to leave blanks. If you really can't work out the answer, it is better to eliminate the answers that you know to be wrong and then make your best guess from those that are left. The answers are multiple-choice and, as the test is not negatively marked, it is better to have a go!

- Throughout the test, there is an option to 'flag' questions. If you are struggling with a question, it is best to have a guess at an answer, flag the question and move on. Then, providing you have time remaining at the end, you can easily identify which questions to return to so that you can work through the question again and amend your answer if necessary. This approach will allow you to secure a reasonable number of marks per section on questions that you are confident with (such as those that are shorter and easier to interpret) before spending time on more complicated questions.

- Be aware that you must read the whole screen of the question that you are on, otherwise you cannot move on to the next question or go back to any of the questions you have answered. There are both vertical and horizontal scroll bars.

- Before you start the test, you should be provided with a mini whiteboard, or as is the case in many test centres, a laminated piece of paper. Since the questions must be completed on a computer, there is no option to highlight or underline key points. In this case, the whiteboard or laminated paper provides a useful tool for jotting down any key points or components of calculations. Do not start the test without one, and if you feel it is necessary, ask for more! With the time pressures of the UCAT, even saving time by not having to rub away answers to previous questions can be incredibly valuable.

- It is worth keeping in mind that the precise scoring method is unknown as it is not information that the UCAT consortium shares. However, it is known that the score you obtain roughly corresponds to the number of questions you answer correctly. A maximum score of 900 is incredibly difficult to obtain, yet it is possible to score 900 and make some mistakes. A competitive score is generally viewed as anything above 700, as this is a difficult score to achieve and exceed.

- Finally, it is most important that you stay calm in the test. Prepare yourself, pace yourself and move on if you're struggling with particular questions. It is inevitable that you will find some questions and some sections easier than others. In the same vein, perspective is important – the UCAT score is one aspect of a series of factors that will enable you to study medicine and is not the single most important part of your application.

Below is a summary of each sub-test, with sample questions provided courtesy of Kaplan Test Prep.

Verbal Reasoning

The Verbal Reasoning test is designed to assess your ability to read and think carefully about information, using comprehension passages to get you to draw specific conclusions from the information presented. The test is based upon the verbal reasoning skills required of doctors to take on board often complex information, to analyse it and then to communicate in simple terms to patients and their families. There are 11 text passages which all have four questions to answer. Some questions will test your comprehension skills by asking you to answer 'true', 'false' or 'can't tell'. In general, if a similar statement can be found in the passage, it is true; if it opposes the information in the text, it is false; and if there is no direct reference to the statement in the passage, we can conclude that we can't tell from the information provided. The other type of question tests your critical response and will look for you to draw a conclusion. You will be presented with an incomplete statement or a question and four response options. You need to pick the most suitable response.

The verbal reasoning section is incredibly challenging, as it requires a rapid pace to get through lengthy passages of text and draw conclusions. In reality, you are unlikely to have much spare time on this section, so it is important to answer each question as you move through, even if it is a guess, rather than wasting time by moving backwards and forwards through questions.

Some candidates prefer to scan-read the passage before reading the questions, as this minimises the time spent reading the questions. Other candidates find this complicated, as it is difficult to remember all of the information in the passage. It may therefore be beneficial to scan-read the statement before looking for phrases relating to it in the passage. It is really important that you practise as many questions as possible, as this will allow you to identify particular strategies that work for you for each question type.

UCAT Verbal Reasoning Practice Questions

Subtest length: 44 questions (11 sets of 4 questions)
Subtest timing: 21 minutes (2 minutes per set)
Sample length: 4 questions
Sample timing: 2 minutes

In 1584, the rediscovery of the works of Tacitus led to the discovery of an old British heroic warrior, Boudicca. No mention is made of Boudicca, also known as Boadicea, in accounts of British history before the Renaissance, but she is referenced in three Roman works: Agricola and The Annals by Tacitus and The Rebellion of Boudicca by

Dio. Thus, since the time of Elizabeth I, another of England's great warrior queens, Boudicca has become a part of England's national history.

Boudicca was the wife of Prasutagus, the head of the Iceni tribe in East England. In the year 43 CE when the Romans invaded England, Prasutagus was one of only two Celtic kings to retain some of his power, and the Romans gave him a grant. The Romans later redefined the grant as a loan, and, when Prasutagus died in 60 CE, he left half of his kingdom to Nero in payment, and the remainder to his daughters. When the Romans came to collect, they seized control of the kingdom, and attacked both Boudicca and her daughters.

Boudicca retaliated by attacking the Roman military's British operational base in Camulodunum, while most of the Roman army was away fighting in Wales. Boudicca's army drove out the Romans and burned Camulodunum to the ground. Boudicca and her army then attacked Londinium; Boudicca had the city burned to the ground and its entire population massacred. The ancient cities of Camulodunum and Londinium were later rebuilt and have since developed into Colchester and London, respectively.

Today, a bronze statue of Boudicca, commissioned during Victoria's reign and unveiled in 1905, stands alongside Westminster Bridge and the Houses of Parliament. The statue carries an inscription from William Cowper's 1782 poem Boadicea, an Ode: 'Regions Caesar never knew / Thy posterity shall sway.' Ironically, England's early anti-imperialist warrior became a primary cultural symbol for the British Empire, and today she stands over the city she once completely destroyed.

1. The British Empire expanded during Victoria's reign.

A.   True
B.   False
C.   Can't tell

2. Following the Roman invasion, Boudicca's husband was allowed to keep some authority over his kingdom.

A.   True
B.   False
C.   Can't tell

3. Roman forces in ancient Britain were headquartered in what is present-day London.

A.   True
B.   False
C.   Can't tell

4. Some Roman historians took note of a foreign warrior queen.

A.   True
B.   False
C.   Can't tell

Decision Making

This test assesses a candidate's ability to apply logic to reach a decision or conclusion, evaluate arguments and analyse statistical information.

A number of skills will be assessed in the decision making element of the UCAT, including:

- deductive reasoning
- evaluating arguments
- statistical reasoning
- figural reasoning.

These skills are assessed through a number of question types:

Logical puzzles

With these questions, you are required to make a deductive inference to arrive at a conclusion. It will involve solving a worded puzzle where some information is given, and the rest you are required to solve. When approaching these questions, you should:

- aim to identify the placement of known facts initially, so that they can be used as a reference for the placement of unknown facts
- eliminate any answers that you know cannot be true
- draw out the information using your whiteboard
- only do the working out that is required – if you do not need to complete the whole puzzle to get the answer, don't waste your time!

Syllogisms

Syllogisms are a form of reasoning where a conclusion is drawn based on a given premise: you are given a statement and asked to draw conclusions based on it. When answering these questions, you should:

- make sure that you have a thorough understanding of the premises given, reading them multiple times if required
- read the conclusions carefully and one by one, so that you can decide whether it is true or false after careful consideration
- avoid making assumptions
- pay attention to the use of qualifying terms.

These questions require a 'drag and drop' response. While it seems straightforward, you should make sure that you spend some time practising this using online practice versions of the test.

Interpreting information

With these questions, information will be presented – the form can vary considerably from passages of text to pie charts – and you must interpret it. You will be expected to draw conclusions based on this information. To increase your chances of getting these questions right, you should:

- try to ignore additional information that is given but is not required
- be prepared to use reasoning skills as opposed to prior knowledge
- where possible, round numbers to solve numerical problems as this will save time calculating
- try not to fall into the trap of basing your answers on the believability of a statement that is made.

Recognising assumptions

In these questions, you will be presented with a number of arguments and you are expected to choose the strongest one. To succeed in these questions, you should:

- ignore your prior beliefs as you must base your responses on the information presented to you
- remember that strong arguments will directly relate to the content in the questions, and this is what you should look out for
- remember assumptions will not be correct, so be careful not to select those as your answer.

Venn diagrams

You will be presented with a Venn diagram and you will be asked to draw conclusions from the information presented within it. You can improve your performance in these questions by:

- revisiting this area of maths and revise it thoroughly
- drawing your own Venn diagram to visualise the answer options.

Probabilistic reasoning

In these questions, you will be given some information containing statistical information and will be required to select the most appropriate response. You should:

- revisit the topic of probability and revise it thoroughly
- eliminate any obviously incorrect statements.

UCAT Decision Making Practice Questions

Subtest length: 29 questions (individual items, rather than sets)
Subtest timing: 31 minutes (1 minute per question)
Sample length: 3 questions
Sample timing: 3 minutes

1. *Vaccine K can prevent 88% of cases of Condition I, but cannot prevent 17% of cases of Condition II.*

Vaccine L cannot prevent 11% of cases of Condition I.

Vaccine L can prevent 86% of cases of Condition II.

Based on the success rates **only**, is Vaccine K more effective than Vaccine L at preventing the conditions?

A.   Yes, because Vaccine K prevents more cases of both conditions.

B.   Yes, because Vaccine K prevents more cases of Condition I than Vaccine L does.

C.   No, because Vaccine L is more successful at preventing both conditions.

D.   No, because Vaccine L is significantly more successful at preventing Condition II, but not Condition I.

2. Should train stations be allowed to charge for the use of the station toilets, which are an essential resource to all passengers who have already paid for a ticket?

Select the strongest argument from the statements below.

A.   Yes, because the cost of cleaning and maintaining the toilets is considerable.

B.   Yes, because most toilets are located in a part of the station that can be accessed by anyone, whether or not they have bought a ticket.

C.   No, because passengers can use the toilets available on the trains.

D.   No, because not everyone uses the toilets in train stations.

3. Some freshwater fish in the minnow family (Cyprinidae), such as the zebrafish, can regenerate their fins, heart or spinal cord following injury or amputation without any mutation or scarring thanks to fibroblast, a specialised protein that acts as a growth factor.

Place 'Yes' if the conclusion does follow. Place 'No' if the conclusion does not follow.

Minnows can regenerate after an injury without any scars.	
If a fish is a freshwater fish, it contains fibroblast.	
Some members of the family Cyprinidae are freshwater fish.	
Zebrafish can survive any injury by regenerating.	
A protein could allow certain minnows to replace an amputated fin	

Quantitative Reasoning

The Quantitative Reasoning test is designed to see if you can solve problems using numerical skills. The test requires you to have good maths skills and knowledge of GCSE level maths. That is not the main point of this test, however; it is more a problem-solving exercise in terms of taking information and manipulating it with calculations and ratios.

As doctors are always using data, it is necessary to test this faculty. From drug calculations to medical research, applicants need to be able to show they have the ability to cope and can respond to different scenarios.

The data will be presented in a variety of ways, including tables, charts and graphs. Not all of the information provided will be immediately obvious, and it will require your close attention to detail to interpret them. Some data sets may not be presented visually at all, and you will be required to pick out the information from passages of text.

While there is some expectation of mathematical ability, you do not have to be exceptionally good at maths to perform well in the quantitative reasoning section. What is more important is being able to identify the appropriate information in the question and avoid making minor errors through carelessness, which is easily done in the time-pressured environment. In fact, some questions may not require you to do any calculations at all, but rather pick out information from visual data such as graphs and pie charts. Many of the calculations are relatively simple, and can be done by estimating.

A major drawback of the numerical reasoning component of the test is that the calculator is on-screen. Practising using an on-screen calculator as you work through questions in preparation is key for familiarising yourself with the process. While it only takes a few seconds longer than using an ordinary calculator, time is of the essence with this section, so any time that can be saved by carrying out calculations mentally will be incredibly valuable!

Sample questions are provided opposite. There are nine sets, each containing four questions, and you will have to choose between five answers. It is a practice-driven section and, as with maths, the more practice you do, the better.

It is worth committing a small proportion of your preparation time to reviewing your knowledge of some key mathematical skills and practising your mental maths so that you are more confident in your approach to more straightforward calculations.

- Being able to convert between percentages and fractions.
- Calculating the area of shapes, e.g. quadrilaterals, triangles and circles.
- Calculating the perimeter of shapes.
- Calculating the circumference of a circle.
- Calculating the volume of an object.
- Calculating percentages.
- Calculating percentage change.

UCAT Quantitative Reasoning Practice Questions

Subtest length: 36 questions (9 sets of 4 questions)
Subtest timing: 24 minutes (2 minutes per set)
Sample length: 4 questions
Sample timing: 2 minutes

The table indicates the total cost of renting different types of helicopter for a particular number of hours. Total cost equals the deposit plus the cost of renting per hour. Some information in the table is missing.

Type	Hours	Deposit	Hourly Rate	Total Cost
A	3	—	£500	£1,680
B	5	£240	£650	—
C	8	—	£4,895	£7,600
D	12	£5,675	£1,100	£13,875

1. Ian's total cost of renting a Type B helicopter was £4,790. For how many hours did he rent the helicopter?

A.   2
B.   3
C.   5
D.   7
E.   9

2. What is the ratio of the total cost of renting a Type A helicopter for 8 hours to the total cost of renting a Type C helicopter for 8 hours?

A.   10:19
B.   11:20
C.   3:5
D.   12:19
E.   8:11

3. The total cost of a Type D helicopter is discounted by a certain rate if rented for 24 hours. Jenni rents a Type D helicopter for 24 hours, with a total cost of £22,743. How much is the discount?

A.   16%
B.   18%
C.   20%
D.   22%
E.   24%

4. Type E helicopters have the same deposit as Type A helicopters. The cost per hour of a Type E helicopter is 25% more than for a Type A helicopter. What is the total cost of renting a Type E helicopter for 6 hours?

A.   £2,430
B.   £2,520
C.   £3,930
D.   £4,080
E.   £4,200

Abstract Reasoning

Abstract Reasoning is designed to assess whether you can look at abstract shapes and then identify patterns, while ignoring the irrelevant material to avoid arriving at the wrong conclusion. What this test aims to do is test whether you are able to change your stance, be critical in your evaluations and create a hypothesis through inquiry.

Patients often give doctors numerous symptoms that doctors have to work through to work out what is relevant and what is not in order to arrive at a diagnosis. Doctors therefore have to use their judgement, as patients are not always accurate in the information they provide.

The patterns that you can be presented with will vary considerably, and some patterns will be far more complex than others. The ability to rapidly identify patterns comes easier to some people than others, but the key is to practise: the more patterns you see and become familiar with, the more readily you will be able to identify them. The abstract reasoning section is the fastest on the whole UCAT exam, so preparation is key!

In the UCAT test, you may see one of four items.

- **Type 1:** two sets of shapes labelled 'Set A' and 'Set B'. From a test shape, you need to decide which set the shape belongs to, or neither.
- **Type 2:** From a series of shapes, you need to select the next shape in the series.
- **Type 3:** A statement will be given about a group of shapes and you then need to conclude which shape would complete the statement.
- **Type 4:** Two sets of shapes will be given to you labelled 'Set A' and 'Set B' and you need to decide from four options which belongs to Set A or Set B.

When approaching abstract reasoning questions, the most important aspect is to identify the pattern in each set. The easiest way of doing this is to pick two shapes – it is advisable to choose the most simplistic – and identify what is common about them. Each set will include shapes that are redundant and play no role in the pattern, so you must get used to ignoring these. For some shapes, there will be one common feature, whereas others may have multiple. These can be to do with the number, size, orientation, positioning and colour of the shapes, as well as the shapes themselves.

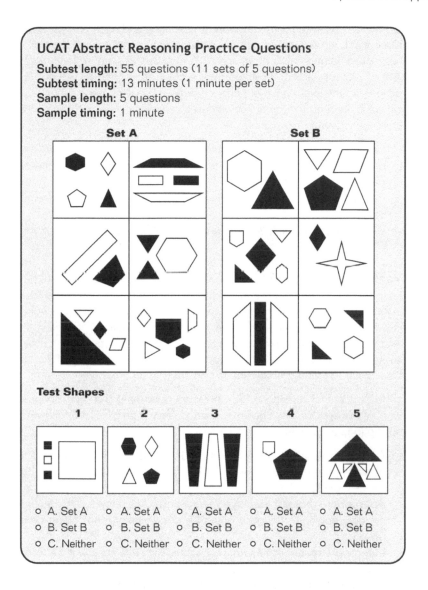

UCAT Abstract Reasoning Practice Questions

Subtest length: 55 questions (11 sets of 5 questions)
Subtest timing: 13 minutes (1 minute per set)
Sample length: 5 questions
Sample timing: 1 minute

Situational Judgement

The Situational Judgement Test is designed to measure how you deal with real-world situations and whether you can identify critical factors and apply appropriate behaviour in the handling of them. What it is ultimately measuring is the level of integrity and perspective you will bring to the profession and whether you are able to work in a multi-disciplinary team.

The score of the Situational Judgement Test is recorded as a 'band', with band 1 representing the highest score and band 4 representing the lowest. These scores are not included in the UCAT average score but are recorded independently and, as such, are typically used separately by medical schools.

You will be presented with 22 different scenarios and each one will have different actions that you could take, with varying considerations. Typically, these considerations will be in line with maintaining a consistently high level of professionalism, having an understanding of medical ethics and recognising the importance of patient safety. There is no expectation that you will have the procedural knowledge to answer these, but it is worth remembering a few key points.

- Under no circumstances should a doctor, or any other medical professional, carry out any action that may affect the confidence of patients in the profession.
- Problems must be addressed as quickly as possible to reassure the patient.
- Where possible, solutions must be identified and put into place efficiently.

The Situational Judgement Test is often viewed as the easiest section, but it should not be underestimated. One reason is that this is the final section of the examination, and you are likely to be fatigued by this point and therefore more likely to make mistakes. In addition, it is a busy section with a large quantity of scenarios in a short period of time. Finally, it may be that each of the possible answers seems plausible, so it is difficult to identify which one is correct.

In the first set of questions, you have to determine the 'appropriateness' of the options in the given scenario. You will be given the following four options to give as your response.

1. **A very appropriate thing to do:** you should give this answer if it addresses at least one aspect of the scenario; it does not have to be all aspects.
2. **Appropriate, but not ideal:** you should give this answer if it was not an ideal solution, though it could be done, despite not being best practice.
3. **Inappropriate, but not awful:** you should give this answer if it should not be done, though it would not be considered terrible.
4. **A very inappropriate thing to do:** you should give this answer if you should definitely not do this.

In giving a response (i.e. 1–4), always remember that it might not be the only course of action and you should not consider it as such.

In the second set, you need to rate the 'importance' of a number of choices regarding a given scenario. You will be given the following four options to give as your response.

1. **Very important:** you would give this answer if this is vital to take into account.
2. **Important:** you would give this answer if it was important but not vital to take into account.

3. **Of minor importance:** you would give this answer if you should take it into account but it would not matter if it was not considered.
4. **Not important at all:** you would give this answer if you should definitely not be taking this information into account.

When approaching these questions, you should consider:

- the appropriateness or importance of the action
- whether the action actually addresses the problem at hand
- whether there are any possible unintended consequences associated with the action.

In addition to the above, the Situational Judgement section has recently introduced a number of scenarios that are answered through a 'drag-and-drop' format: each question has multiple components and you must drag the correct answer and drop it into each component.

UCAT Situational Judgement Practice Questions

Subtest length: 20 scenarios, 2 to 5 questions each (69 questions total)
Subtest timing: 26 minutes (20–30 seconds per scenario, then 10–15 seconds per question)
Sample length: 4 questions
Sample timing: 1 minute

A medical student, Emmet, is completing a patient history as part of his placement at a GP surgery. The patient has previously been treated for emphysema and has difficulty breathing, but he has continued to smoke. The patient mentions that the doctor 'keeps telling me to quit' but insists that he enjoys cigarettes, they help him to relax, and 'you're not taking away my one pleasure in life'. Emmet has experience as a volunteer on a stop smoking campaign, so he feels qualified to engage with the patient on this issue.

How **appropriate** are each of the following responses by Emmet in this situation?

1. Discuss other relaxing activities, such as reading, music or sport, that the patient might enjoy.

A.   A very appropriate thing to do

B.   Appropriate, but not ideal

C.   Inappropriate, but not awful

D.   A very inappropriate thing to do

2. Tell the patient that he risks shortening his life, with reduced quality of life, if he keeps smoking.

A.   A very appropriate thing to do

B.   Appropriate, but not ideal

C.   Inappropriate, but not awful

D.   A very inappropriate thing to do

3. Remind the patient that the doctors know best and he would do well to follow their advice.

A.   A very appropriate thing to do

B.   Appropriate, but not ideal

C.   Inappropriate, but not awful

D.   A very inappropriate thing to do

Verbal Reasoning Practice Questions - Answers

1. (C)

2. (A)

3. (B)

4. (A)

Decision Making Practice Questions - Answers

1. (C)

2. (B)

3. NO; NO; YES; NO; YES

Quantitative Reasoning Practice Questions - Answers

1. (D)

2. (B)

3. (A)

4. (C)

Abstract Reasoning Practice Questions - Answers

1. (A)

2. (C)

3. (C)

4. (A)

5. (B)

Situational Judgement Practice Questions - Answers

1. (A)

2. (B)

3. (D)

All practice questions provided by Kaplan Test Prep, a leading provider of preparation for the UCAT and BMAT. See www.kaptest.com/ucat to learn more about preparing with Kaplan Test Prep.

How do universities use the UCAT?

The utilisation of UCAT scores varies considerably between the different medical schools, and the guidance tends to change slightly each year. It is therefore crucial that the information provided here is utilised alongside that on the websites of the medical schools, as well as the information provided by the UCAT consortium.

If you have underperformed in the UCAT, obtaining an average score of less than the average, which is typically around 630, it is not the end of the road for your medicine application. You should focus on universities that put more weighting in the selection process on other aspects of your application, and so do not focus on the UCAT score quite as much. These universities include:

- Cardiff University, which ranks applicants based on their academic performance, using the UCAT score only in borderline cases
- Keele University, which has a low cut-off score (2280 overall score for 2020 entry)
- University of Plymouth, which has a low cut-off score (2400 for 2021 entry).

Below are some examples of the ways in which the UCAT was used by medical schools for 2019 entry.

University of Birmingham

There is no minimum UCAT cut-off score. Your total UCAT score from the four subtests (i.e. excluding the band result for the Situational Judgement Test, SJT), will be ranked among those for all applicants. The scores will be segregated into deciles and we will allocate our own score to each decile. For example, the top 10% of applicants' scores will be in the top decile and will receive a maximum score of 3.0 in our process. For guidance, the decile ranges in 2019–20 were as follows (converted to a 0–3 scale):

Table 5 UCAT

Total UCAT score	Decile	Converted score
2910 and above	10th	3.000
2790–2900	9th	2.667
2730–2780	8th	2.333
2670–2720	7th	2.000
2620–2660	6th	1.667
2560–2610	5th	1.333
2500–2550	4th	1.000
2420–2490	3rd	0.667
2320–2410	2nd	0.333
2310 and below	1st	0.000

It is important to note that the thresholds for each decile will be different for a new set of applicants. Therefore, the UCAT score applied to your application may differ from the above table but the difference is expected to be marginal. The decile boundaries for 2018–19 were very similar to those in Table 5 (page 75), therefore we expect your UCAT score will fall either in the decile indicated above or in an adjacent decile.

University of Bristol

All applicants are required to take the UCAT in the current cycle. The combined score from all sub-tests, with the exception of Situational Judgement, will be used to select applicants for interview. For 2019 entry, applicants with a UCAT score of 2730 or above were invited to interview. However, the number used as a threshold for interview is subject to change year-on-year.

University of East Anglia

All applicants are required to take the UCAT in the year of application, prior to applying. UEA does not have a cut-off score. A high score is advantageous; however, a low score does not disqualify an applicant from consideration. The subsection scores may be used to rank the applicants for selection for interview. The overall score is used alongside the interview score to rank and select applicants to whom an offer is made. The SJT component score is included within the interview score.

The Situational Judgement Test

Although most students focus on the average UCAT score consideration of medical schools, many schools now also look at performance on the SJT.

Several universities do not consider performance on the SJT at all. At the time of writing, these include:

- University of Aberdeen (but it may be used in offer-making when there are candidates with similar scores)
- University of Bristol
- University of Dundee (but Band 4 may affect the decision on whether or not to make an offer)
- University of Glasgow
- University of Plymouth
- Queen's University Belfast
- University of Southampton
- St George's, University of London.

Medical schools that do use the SJT tend to only do so in the case of obtaining a Band 4, which results in rejection. These universities include:

- Anglia Ruskin University
- Edge Hill University

- University of Edinburgh
- Keele University
- University of Leicester
- University of Lincoln
- University of Liverpool (with the exception of international applicants)
- Newcastle University
- University of Nottingham
- University of Manchester
- University of Sunderland.

A number of universities, including Cardiff University, the University of Exeter and Aston University, do not provide any formal guidance on how the SJT is used. While it is most likely to be the case that it is not used, it is worth approaching these universities with caution in the case of a poor SJT score.

As well as being used to make outright decisions, performance in the SJT can also influence whether or not you are invited to interview. The following universities demonstrate a specific scoring mechanism whereby the SJT score contributes:

- University of Edinburgh
- Hull York Medical School
- King's College, London
- University of Lincoln
- University of Nottingham.

Similarly, the SJT can also influence the interview process directly. In some cases, a high SJT score would place you at an advantage at the interview stage, even if it did not contribute to getting you the interview in the first place. Medical schools that will scrutinise applicants with a low SJT score more heavily at interview include:

- University of East Anglia
- University of Birmingham
- Hull York Medical School
- Queen Mary University of London
- University of Sheffield
- University of St Andrews.

It is important to note that this information is accurate at the time of writing, but you should always check with each individual university to ensure that their stance regarding the importance of the SJT has not changed.

UCAT fees

- Test taken in the UK/EU: £75
- Test taken in the EU: £120

This information is accurate at the time of writing, but will be updated in April 2021 for 2022 applications.

UCAT SJTace

The Situational Judgement Test for Admission to Clinical Education was taken up for 2018/19 by the universities of Dundee and St Andrews for their Scottish Graduate Entry Medical (ScotGEM) programme. It is designed to select the candidates who they deem to have the right professional behaviour necessary to be successful in the medical profession. It is identical to the Situational Judgement Test in the standard UCAT test.

BMAT (BioMedical Admissions Test)

The BMAT is a test to ensure effective selection of well-qualified students. At present, 32 medical schools use this test (as outlined in Table 6, below) though only nine are UK universities. This is a written test and is deemed a productive indicator of a student's likely result in their first year of undergraduate study.

Table 6 Medical schools requiring BMAT admissions test

Medical school	UCAS course code
Brighton and Sussex Medical School	A100
Imperial College London	A100, A109
Lancaster University	A100, A900
University College London	A100
University of Cambridge	A100
University of Leeds	A100
University of Manchester (for some international students only)	A106, A104
University of Oxford	A100
Keele University (for international students)	A100
University of Rijeka, Croatia	Medicine
University of Zagreb, Croatia	Doctor of Medicine (in English)
Universita Campus BioMedico di Roma (UCBM), Italy	MD Program in Medicine and Surgery (for non-European citizens not resident in Italy)
University of Pécs, Hungary	Medicine
Nazarbayev University School of Medicine, Kazakhstan	MD (Postgraduate Medicine)
Leiden University Medical Centre (LUMC), The Netherlands	Medicine
Medical University Warsaw, Poland	MD programme in English
Pomeranian Medical University in Szczecin, Poland	MD programme in English

Vasile Goldis Western university of Arad, Romania	Medicine (in English)
CEU Cardenal Herrera University, Spain	Medicine
Universidad de Navarra, Spain	Medicine
Pirogov Russian National Research Medical University, Moscow, Russia	General Medicine
University of Malaya, Malaysia	Doctor of Medicine
Chiang Mai University, Thailand	Doctor of Medicine
Chulalongkorn University, Thailand	Doctor of Medicine
Khon Kaen University, Thailand	MD02 Medicine (Northeast Thailand applicants), MDX Medicine (other applicants)
King Mongkut's Institute of Technology, Ladkrabang, Thailand	Medicine
Mahidol University, Thailand	Medicine
Navamindradhiraj University, Thailand	MD Doctor of Medicine
Srinakharinwirot University, Thailand	A105, MD Doctor of Medicine
Suranaree University of Technology, Thailand	MD Doctor of Medicine
Thammasat University: CICM and Dentistry, Thailand	624901 Doctor of Medicine (English language)
Lee Kong Chian School of Medicine, Singapore	Medicine

All candidates applying to institutions or courses in Table 6 above are required to take the BMAT. The test, which takes place in November (usually in your school), consists of three sections. In previous years, it has also been possible to sit the test in September (for a higher fee), though due to the Covid-19 pandemic, the September series was cancelled in 2020. It is yet to be determined whether this test will be reinstated for 2021. All important dates regarding the BMAT exam can be found at www.bmat.org.uk.

The test can only be taken once per cycle, and many students opt to take the BMAT at the later November date to allow for more preparation time. However, by sitting the BMAT in September (providing this is an option) you will be able to make more informed decisions about your university choices, since you will have the score prior to the UCAS deadline.

Sample questions for each section are included below, courtesy of Kaplan Test Prep.

1. **Thinking skills:** such as problem solving, understanding arguments, data analysis, critical thinking, logic and reasoning (60 minutes; 32 multiple-choice or short-answer questions).

BMAT® Thinking Skills Practice Questions

Have a go at the below sample BMAT Thinking Skills practice questions, taken from the full set.

DIRECTIONS (for full test):

Answer every question. Points are awarded for correct answers only. There are no penalties for incorrect answers. All questions are worth 1 mark.

3. The media frequently shares stories about the supposed dangers of screen time for children and teenagers, but there has been little discussion of the appropriate amount of screen time for adults. Recent research indicates that adults average 11 hours of screen time per day, which means that adults spend most of our waking time looking at screens. That figure has increased from nine and a half hours four years ago. Of the current figures, 43% of daily screen time is spent watching TV, 21% using smartphones, and 7% using tablets. This data underlines the fact that concerns about people spending too much time looking at smartphones are misguided, since adults actually spend significantly more time watching TV.

Which of the following is the best statement of the conclusion in the argument above?

A No one can say how much daily screen time is suitable for adults.

B It is unwarranted to worry that someone's smartphone screen time is excessive.

C Compared to smartphone usage, watching TV takes up more of the average adult's day.

D Adults spend more and more time looking at screens each year.

E There is not enough awareness of the dangers of screen time for adults.

4. The clocks in Beematia use an unusual format to indicate the time. Beematia uses a 24-hour clock in the format mm:hh, in which mm indicates the number of minutes to the next hour (hh). For example, 12:05 indicates the time is 12 minutes before 5am. Each day in Beematia has 24 hours and each hour has 60 minutes.

Srinand is visiting Beematia, and the clocks in his hotel room indicate the time in this format.

The clock in the hotel room says 19:22 when Srinand goes to sleep. When he wakes up, the clock reads 22:07.

For how long has Srinand slept?

A 2 hours, 45 minutes

B 7 hours, 41 minutes

C 8 hours, 57 minutes

D 9 hours, 3 minutes

E 10 hours, 19 minutes

Answers

3. B

4. C

2. **Scientific knowledge and applications:** the ability to apply scientific knowledge, from school science to maths (30 minutes; 27 multiple-choice or short-answer questions). You are tested on your core knowledge and whether you have the capacity to apply it – key for high level biomedical sciences. The questions you will have are related to material that would have been included 'in non-specialist school science and maths courses'. You therefore have to have a good level of understanding in these subjects. Questions are multiple-choice and calculators may not be used. Biology, chemistry and physics all carry eight marks each and maths carries six marks.

BMAT® Scientific Knowledge and Applications Practice Questions

Have a go at the below sample BMAT Scientific Knowledge and Applications practice questions, taken from the full set.

DIRECTIONS (for full test):

Answer every question. Points are awarded for correct answers only. There are no penalties for incorrect answers. All questions are worth 1 mark. Some questions have more than 1 correct answer. Read carefully to ensure that you select the appropriate number of answers. Calculators are not permitted during any portion of the test.

1. Freckles are autosomal dominant, meaning that a child with at least one dominant allele will have freckles. Children with a recessive genotype will not have freckles.

A husband and wife both have freckles, but their first child does not have freckles.

What is the probability that their next child will have freckles?

A 0%

B 12.5%

C 25%

D 37.5%

E 50%

F 62.5%

G 75%

H 100%

3. The first five hexagonal numbers are 1, 6, 15, 28 and 45.

The difference between the first and second hexagonal numbers is 5.

The difference between the second and third hexagonal numbers is 9.

The difference between the third and fourth hexagonal numbers is 13.

The difference between the fourth and fifth hexagonal numbers is 17.

All the hexagonal numbers follow this pattern.

The difference between the rth hexagonal number and the $(r + 3)$th hexagonal number is 363.

What is the value of r?

A 28

B 29

C 30

D 31

E 32

Answers

1. G

3. B

3. **Writing task:** this tests your ability to select, develop and organise ideas and to communicate them in writing, concisely and effectively. You must complete one essay question from a choice of three, which requires you to construct an argument or a debate, analyse a statement or a similar yet equal-based task (30 minutes; one from a choice of three short essay questions). You have a choice from a selection of tasks and one must be selected. These will include brief questions based on topics of general and medical interest. The questions require you to explain or discuss the proposition's implications, propose counter arguments and identify resolutions. This is your opportunity to demonstrate effective written communication. Marks are awarded based on addressing the question in the way it is required, clarity of thought and concise expression.

BMAT® Writing Practice Questions

Time: 30 minutes

Have a go at the writing practice questions, taken from the full set. Here we show two of the four essay title options.

DIRECTIONS (for full test):

Answer only one task from the choice of four essay titles. You must write your answer by hand, and are limited to a space consisting of one side of A4. You are permitted to make any preparatory notes as needed, but time spent on such notes counts against the 30 minutes allowed for the essay. In this task, you are expected to show how well you can order and explore ideas, and convey these ideas in clear, effective writing. You may not use dictionaries or any other reference books or resources. Essays are assigned a numerical score. To achieve a top mark, you must address all aspects of the question and write compellingly with few errors in logic or in use of English.

1. **All 16-year-olds should be required to complete first aid training, as part of the National Curriculum.**

Write an essay in which you address the following points:

What are the advantages in training all 16-year-olds in how to give CPR and deal with heart attacks, strokes and other major injuries? What are the drawbacks of requiring such training? To what extent do you agree that some first aid training should be compulsory, and at what age?

2. **Research is what I'm doing when I don't know what I'm doing.**
(Wernher von Braun, German scientist, 1912–1977)

Write an essay in which you address the following points:

Explain what this statement means. Argue that a scientist can only undertake research with a clear goal or objective in mind. To what extent do you agree with von Braun that research is possible, or preferable, when scientists don't know what they're doing?

All practice questions provided by Kaplan Test Prep, a leading provider of preparation for the UCAT and BMAT. See www.kaptest.com/bmat to learn more about preparing with Kaplan Test Prep.

In Sections 1 and 2, points are scored on a nine-point scale to one decimal place. In Section 3, marks are awarded based on quality of content and quality of written English (A, B or C) and placed on a five-point scale out of 5. The written task is marked by the Admissions Testing Service.

For 2020 exams, Section 1 was updated so that it did not include questions that test data analysis and inference. In previous years, students have had to complete questions that assess whether they can understand verbal, statistical and graphical information. It is assumed that this update will remain in place for 2021.

Unlike the UCAT, you cannot use calculators or dictionaries, including bilingual dictionaries, in the exam. Similarly, it is also possible to prepare more thoroughly for the BMAT: there is a specification that is accessible, and revision can be conducted for each section, especially Section 2. In addition, there are vast quantities of past paper questions available along with mark schemes for you to familiarise yourself with the level of questioning in the exam.

Guidance on marks

- **Brighton and Sussex Medical School:** The BMAT is scored out of 28, which is a total from all three elements and an extra five marks on the essay for good use of English language, making the essay very important to the process. In 2019, applicants who scored 16.1 or above were invited to interview. Without contextual data, students who did not score at least 3 on Section 1 and 2, as well as 2.5C on Section 3, were not considered
- **University of Oxford:** The average BMAT score for successful applicants has been around 63.5% historically, and 62% for those invited to interview. They primarily focus on Sections 1 and 2, which contribute 40% each, with the remaining 20% focusing on Section 3.
- **University of Cambridge:** While Oxford uses a centralised system, Cambridge uses its collegiate system when assessing BMAT scores, which means there is no general guidance. Historically, offer holders have secured high grades of above 6 (out of 9) on Sections 1 and 2, and over 3 (out of 5) for Section 3.
- **Imperial College London:** Imperial is unique in that it is still the only university to have a cut-off score across three sections. If candidates do not secure these scores, they will not be shortlisted for interview. In 2019, Home/EU candidates were required to score a minimum of 4.1 in Section 1 and 4.2 in Section 2; they were required to score a minimum of 2.5C in Section 3. Overseas candidates were required to score a minimum of 4.0 in Section 1 and Section 2, with the sum of scores in these two Sections being at least 10.0; they were required to score a minimum of 3C in Section 3.
- **University of Leeds:** Leeds uses the BMAT score as part of an overall scoring process alongside academic attainment and the personal statement.
- **University of Lancaster:** The BMAT is scored out of 13, a total of all three elements. In 2019, students with a BMAT score of 9.3 or above were interviewed (meaning you need to achieve, roughly, a minimum of 4.0 in Sections 1 and 2, and 2.5 in Section 3).
- **University College London:** A good BMAT result is helpful to your application to UCL, though it is important to remember that it is not the only factor. In previous years, the average scores of interviewees were 5.3 out of 9 for Sections 1 and 2, and 3.3 out of 5 for Section 3.

General hints

- Familiarity with the basic structure of the test is good preparation, so make sure that you utilise the past paper questions available on the website. This is especially useful for Section 1, which requires the development of skills for the aptitude test.
- You can revise for Section 2 of the test as it covers biology, chemistry, physics and maths to GCSE standard.
- As with the UCAT, the majority of candidates do not complete all sections in the test so don't worry if you don't. Ensure that you have tried the practice tests first so that you understand the timing of the test. Try to answer as many questions as you can but do not worry if you do not get to the end of each section. If you are short on time, make sure that you do not leave an answer blank – the test is not negatively marked, so it is worth having a go!
- Practise writing the essays under timed conditions and using BMAT test paper, since there is a space constraint. Where possible, get advice from a teacher about how best to structure your essays and make best use of the time and space available.
- You can access a specification for the BMAT exam, so it is advisable that you review this carefully as part of your preparation.
- In Sections 1 and 2, there is a point for each right answer, but no points are deducted for wrong answers.
- In Section 3, each of the essays is double marked and there is a mark for the quality of written English presentation.
- It might be obvious, but the best thing you can do is stay calm. If you have put in the time to practise beforehand, then you have prepared as best you can. Do not ruin your chances by letting nerves get in your way.

5 | The personal statement

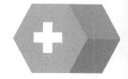

'How important is the personal statement? It gets the foot in the door. Without a good personal statement, you may not progress to the other stages where you will shine.'

Dr Vicki Cooney; practising GP, London

One of the most important parts of your application is your personal statement, as this is your chance to show the university selectors three very important themes. These are:

- why you want to be a doctor
- what you have done to investigate the profession
- whether you are the right sort of person for their medical school (in other words, the personal qualities that make you an outstanding candidate).

The personal statement is your opportunity to demonstrate to the admissions tutors not only that you have researched medicine thoroughly, but that you also have the right personal qualities to succeed as a doctor, you are fully committed to studying medicine and have the right motivation and personal qualities to do so successfully. A typical personal statement takes time and effort to get right; don't expect perfection after one draft.

When it comes to distinguishing between highly qualified candidates, one of the most important factors that is considered is the personal statement. If this is badly worded, littered with errors or lacking detail about the attributes and experiences of the candidate, it will stand a chance of being rejected without being taken further. Ultimately, this means that the more thought that you give to your UCAS application and personal statement, the better they will be and the greater your chance of being asked to come in for an interview and being made a conditional offer.

Another important consideration is the fact that your personal statement needs to be no more than 47 lines long or 4,000 characters (including spaces); this is a strict limit and so you need to ensure that you are as close to this as possible.

Sections of the personal statement

Why medicine?

Your personal statement must, fundamentally, convince admissions tutors of your interest in following a career in medicine.

A high proportion of UCAS applications contain a sentence like 'From an early age I have wanted to be a doctor because it is the only career that combines my love of science with the chance to work with people.' Not only do admissions tutors get bored with reading this, it doesn't necessarily highlight your desire to study medicine: there are many careers that combine science and people, including teaching, pharmacy, physiotherapy and nursing.

However, the basic ideas behind this sentence may well apply to you. If so, you need to personalise it. You could mention an incident that first got you interested in medicine – a visit to your own doctor, a conversation with a family friend, or a lecture at school, for instance. You could write about your interest in human biology or a biology project that you undertook when you were younger to illustrate your interest in science, and you could give examples of how you like to work with others. The important thing is to back up your initial interest with your efforts to investigate the career.

It is a common misconception that you need to begin your personal statement with an inspirational quotation or grand statement; again, admissions tutors get bored of students trying to squeeze in lines from books, poems or films that have no real meaning to the applicant. What an admissions tutor would rather see is a statement of the genuine reasons that you want to study medicine, written in clear, uncomplicated English.

Another common pitfall in the first paragraph is taking up valuable space with an explanation about what the subject is about or what the profession entails. For example: 'Medicine is a highly regarded profession that involves the diagnosis, treatment and prevention of disease.' Remember that the people reading your statement know exactly what the profession is about and so do not need to be lectured on it! Instead, you need to take the time to explain about your own interest in the profession and why you feel compelled to follow this career path.

Finally, don't be afraid to lean on your work experience placements or voluntary work here. Often, those initial sparks of interest in a career in medicine are underpinned by what you observed when shadowing a doctor in A&E, or when you were playing board games with elderly patients in a care home. This section of the personal statement should be sizeable, so it is a good idea to link your motivation to study medicine in with your experiences of healthcare. These experiences will also form a significant proportion of your personal statement.

Work experience and voluntary work

This section is important to demonstrate that you gained something from your work experience and voluntary placements, and that they have given you an insight into the profession. Start by talking about your medicine-specific experiences. You should give an indication of the length of time you spent at each placement and the impressions you gained. You could comment on what aspects of medicine attract you, or on what you found interesting or something that you hadn't expected, but remember that this is not a shopping list. You are not simply reeling off experience after experience; you are expected to provide deeper reflection about what you have seen. Beyond this, you should also mention any other work experience or voluntary work you have had in a caring or clinical role and what you learned from it. Although you may not think of these sorts of experiences as being relevant, they can often demonstrate to an admissions tutor good interpersonal skills or commitment and dedication, all of which are relevant to medicine.

Here is a sample description of a student's work experience that would probably not impress the admissions team.

> 'I spent three days at my local GP surgery. I saw a patient have their blood pressure taken. It was very interesting.'

In contrast, the example below would be much more convincing because it is clear that the student was interested in what was happening.

> 'During a two-week placement at my local GP surgery, I shadowed two GPs and a clinical nurse. As well as being able to observe how the doctors and nurses interacted with anxious and unwell patients, I was able to witness a number of medical interventions, including blood samples being taken, blood pressure being measured and a referral recommendation to a specialist doctor following a patient's complaints of back pain. What I found particularly interesting was the fact that, although both doctors had very different personalities, they both related well to the patients, who seemed to find them very reassuring. A number of things surprised me; in particular, how varying a doctor's day can be.'

Spelling mistakes, grammatical errors and unclear personal statements will create an unfavourable impression on the selectors. In order to ensure that this does not happen, follow these tips.

It will be far easier to write this section of your personal statement if you kept notes in a reflective journal during your work experience as discussed previously. Look back over what you wrote and use your thoughts and experiences as a stimulus for this section. With luck, the admissions tutors may pick up on these experiences at interview and ask you to expand on some of your comments.

Following this, you should discuss the experiences you have had whilst undertaking any voluntary work. Any type of voluntary placement is a useful addition to your statement, but ongoing work in a care-based or clinical setting really boosts your profile. Opportunities often exist in care homes, children's hospices and hospitals and it is worth trying to contribute regularly over a long period of time rather than carrying it out for just a week or two. This type of experience can help you get an insight into patient care and the communication side of the profession and gives a really good opportunity to discuss how your interpersonal skills have developed whilst working with people. As with any medical work experience, you should make a note of any key experiences that you have and what they have taught you, as this can then be commented on in your personal statement.

With Covid-19, there is an understanding from medical schools that you may not have been able to carry out work experience or voluntary work as planned. The important thing to remember is that admissions tutors are looking for a thorough understanding of the medical professional and what the role of a doctor entails. This can be achieved through talking to medical students, doctors and other healthcare professionals, online research (including social media, blogs and vlogs), online learning (such as free courses), keeping an eye on the news and even virtual work experience opportunities. There might also be voluntary roles that you could take on in your local area to enhance your application. Further information about how to gain an insight into the profession in a pandemic can be found in Chapter 2.

Your academic interests

It is important for your personal statement to contain information about your academic interests and how they have furthered your desire to study medicine. This may be related to some topics or practical skills that have been of particular interest to you over the course of your A level studies, or to an interesting article you have read in a newspaper or journal, or to something engaging you heard in a lecture. Whatever it is, it will help to demonstrate your desire to pursue the course, as long as you make it relevant to medicine and put in sufficient detail. In so many personal statements this section struggles to get beyond 'I enjoyed learning about the human body' and 'I enjoy using different apparatus in practical work'; however, this is too generic to be meaningful. Keeping a journal over a long period of time of any wider reading that is relevant to medicine will help this section to genuinely reflect what your interests are rather than being based on what you have panic-read the week before submitting your application.

Evidence of developing skills and personal qualities

The person reading your UCAS application has to decide two things: whether you have the right skills and personal qualities to become a successful doctor, and whether you will be able to cope with and contribute to medical school life. To be a successful medic, you need (among other things!) to:

- successfully pass your undergraduate studies
- have good interpersonal skills and get on with a wide range of people
- be able to work under pressure and cope with stress
- have well-developed manual skills.

How, then, does the person reading your personal statement know whether you have the qualities they are looking for? What you must remember is that the admissions tutor doesn't know you, so you have to give lots of evidence of how you have demonstrated and developed these qualities. Some of the things they may be looking for are:

- skill development during work experience/voluntary work
- positions of responsibility
- work in the local community
- an ability to get on with people
- participation in activities involving manual dexterity
- participation in team events
- involvement in school plays or concerts.

Some examples of aspects that you might want to include in your application are detailed below.

Have you demonstrated a range of interests?

Medical schools like to see applicants who have done more with their life than work for their A levels and watch TV. While the teacher writing your reference will probably refer to your outstanding academic achievements, you also need to say something about your achievements in your personal statement. Admissions tutors like to read about achievements in sport and other outdoor activities, such as the Duke of Edinburgh's Award Scheme. Equally useful activities include Young Enterprise, charity work, public speaking, part-time jobs, art, music and drama.

Bear in mind that admissions tutors will be asking themselves: 'Would this person be an asset to the medical school?' Put in enough detail and try to make it interesting to read. An important point to note though is that extra-curricular information must not take up more than about 25% of your personal statement, as the primary focus is on why you want to get in to medicine.

The key is to ensure that you are always relating your personal qualities and extra-curricular activities to your application, in order to show evidence of the attributes and skills needed to become a doctor. It needs to be relevant to the medical application, to demonstrate to admission tutors that you are the right sort of person for the university.

Here is an example of a good paragraph on interests for the personal statement section:

'I very much enjoy tennis and play in the school team and for Hampshire at under-18 level. This summer a local sports shop has sponsored me to attend a tennis camp in California. I worked at the Wimbledon championships in 2016. Doing so has placed the emphasis of team work and personal reliance on me. I have been playing the piano since the age of eight and took my Grade 7 exam recently, which I think demonstrates manual dexterity. At school, I play in the orchestra and in a very informal jazz band. Last year I started learning the trombone but I would not like anyone except my teacher to hear me playing! Music is a perfect way to relax; at the same time, it got me thinking about the link between music and medicine. The discipline and dedication of years of practice required in both is similar – not to mention the manual dexterity integral in each – but more so, looking into it, I have become fascinated by the link between the two, both from a therapeutic perspective – music therapy for example being a new technique designed to interact with patients – and a relaxation standpoint; anything from the music in a doctor's waiting room to the music playing in an operating room to calm the surgeon and help them focus. I like dancing and social events but my main form of relaxation is gardening. I have started a small business helping my neighbours to improve their gardens – which also brings in some extra money.'

And here's how not to do it:

'I play tennis in competitions and the piano and trombone. I like gardening.'

But what if you aren't musical, can't play tennis and find geraniums boring? It depends when you are reading this. Anyone with enough drive to become a doctor can probably rustle up an interest or two in six months. If you haven't even got that long, then it would be sensible to devote most of your personal statement to your interest in medicine.

Have you contributed to school activities?
This is largely covered by the section on interests, but it is worth noting that the selector is looking for someone who will contribute to the communal life of the medical school. If you have been involved in organising things in your school, do remember to include the details. Don't forget to say that you ran the school's fundraising barbecue or that you organised guest speakers for the college medical society. Conversely, medical schools are less interested in applicants whose activities are exclusively solitary or cannot take place in the medical school environment.

The admissions tutors will be aware that some schools offer more to their students in the way of activities and responsibilities than others. However, even if there are very few opportunities made available to you through your school, you must still find ways to gain experience and develop your skills. You don't have to have been captain of the rugby team or gone on a three-month expedition to Borneo to be considered, but you do need to be able to demonstrate that you have made efforts to participate in a range of worthwhile activities.

Have you any achievements or leadership experience to your credit?

Admissions tutors are particularly attracted by excellence in any sphere. Have you competed in any activity at a high level or received a prize or other recognition for your achievements? Have you organised and led any events or team games? Were you elected as class representative to the school council? If so, make sure that you include it in your personal statement.

WARNING!

- Don't copy any of the paragraphs above on to your own UCAS application.
- Don't write anything that isn't true.
- Don't write anything you can't talk about at the interview.
- Avoid over-complicated, over-formal styles of writing. Read your personal statement out loud; if it doesn't sound like you speaking, rewrite it.

TIP!

Keep a copy of your personal statement so that you can look at it when you prepare for the interview.

Things to avoid

Writing your personal statement can be a difficult and long-winded process. There are some things easy to avoid that will ensure that you make a good impression with your application.

1. **Not enough words.**

   You must ensure that the personal statement is as close to the 4,000 character limit as possible. Anything significantly below the character count will make a negative impression on the admissions tutors.

2. **A lack of detail or reflection.**

   It is crucial that you do not simply list your experiences, but carefully reflect on them to ensure that the admissions tutors can see that you have gained a lot from them. When discussing work experience, go into detail about what you witnessed and reflect on what you learned. When giving details of what you are studying, be specific about topics you have enjoyed. This will give the admissions tutor a much greater insight into who you are and the skills you possess.

3. **Not being very personal.**
   Make sure your personal statement has evidence and experiences to show an admissions tutor who you really are and what you are genuinely interested in.

4. **Negativity.**
   Unfortunately, many personal statements contain negative points about things that an applicant hasn't enjoyed studying or things they might not like about the career. These are sometimes included due to a misguided need to be brutally honest, but this really is not necessary. The overall tone should be optimistic and positive throughout.

5. **Lecturing about medicine.**
   Statements can often waste time by listing facts about medicine or what doctors do. Remember that the people reading your statement will know all of this. Use the space instead to illustrate from your own experiences that you possess the qualities and skills that doctors need.

6. **Discussing money and potential earnings.**
   Although most medicine applicants will have thought about how much money they will be making at some point, it is not something that needs to be highlighted in your personal statement. Your reasons for studying medicine need to run much deeper than this if you are going to get into medical school.

7. **The use of overused, repeated stock phrases.**
   Commonly used statements can make an admissions tutor question whether your statement is an accurate picture of who you are. If you genuinely want to express a generic idea, think of how you could expand on it in your own words to make it more meaningful.

8. **Losing the focus on medicine.**
   If the only place that really comes alive in your personal statement is when you are discussing how much you enjoy studying English Literature, then you are misusing the space that you have available. Transfer that enthusiasm to elements of your personal statement that the admissions tutors will want to see.

9. **Overusing the thesaurus.**
   Beware of overusing a thesaurus. Obviously, you want your English to be as good as possible, but make sure that what you have written makes sense and sounds like you.

Four sample statements can be found on the following pages. The examples demonstrate clarity and focus, and what comes through the most is the enthusiasm that the candidates have for medicine. These attributes will give an applicant an excellent chance of being called in for an interview and/or just being given an offer.

Personal statement: Example 1 (character count: 3,991)

Studying medicine, to me, is the perfect blend of my keen interest in human biology with the invaluable opportunity of working to improve the lives of others. Through exploring career options, speaking to medics and doing work experience, I am inspired to pursue medicine as it results in a stimulating career path.

Volunteering at the Sunrise of Solihull care home for a year has increased my determination to study medicine. Here, I learnt the value of empathy, when a resident with dementia became agitated under my care. This was overwhelming and encouraged me to learn more by reading *Memory's Last Breath: Field Notes on my Dementia*. The memoir gave me an insight into the biological nature of microvascular disease as a cause of dementia. Gaining an indepth understanding of the resident's behaviour enabled me to empathise with her and adapt the way I spoke to her. Building up a rapport between us, and thus reducing her anxiety, was extremely satisfying. This has inspired me to undertake an EPQ in my gap year to explore more about dementia.

During my work experience at a local general practice, I observed how the GP comforted a woman with chronic pain syndrome sensitively within immense time pressures. The way he supported the patient, in addition to decision making in a non-judgemental manner, urged me to critique my management skills. While volunteering with Solihull Life Opportunities for a year, I was able to plan activity days and execute them to a group of children with various disabilities. Spending time with the children was eye opening as I saw how, despite their various illnesses, they never lacked positivity. This was inspiring, and the idea of contributing to a community that can support both patients and their families gratifies me. I spent a day helping the receptionists at the general practice. I saw how they handled the demands of the public in a respectful way using valuable communication skills. In order to develop my verbal and non-verbal communication skills, I took part in leading a summer camp for children at my local temple, which received good feedback.

I observed how doctors work in a multidisciplinary team when I spent a week doing work experience at Walsgrave Hospital. The endoscopy team had to deal with an unexpected bleed due to polyps in the bowel, and it was amazing to see how confidently they managed it. I observed the consultant making decisions, taking responsibility for his actions and leading the team, with confidence and resilience, in order to save a life. These are skills I continue to develop through my participation in activities in and out of school.

At school, I led the Religious Studies club, where I organised discussions about ethical issues such as abortion and euthanasia. Through studying psychology and religious studies alongside my chemistry and biology A levels, I have been able to gain a broader understanding of human behaviours and ethics. Being a form mentor and organising revision sessions for GCSE students has developed my organisational skills. I regularly participated in my school's medical society where I made a presentation on notable women in the field of medicine.

I have been playing the drums for seven years, and as a member of a band, I value the role of teamwork, as it is imperative for a successful performance. I will continue to develop my drumming skills during my gap year and work towards my grade 8 examination. Being a team leader at the National Citizens Service, delegating tasks fairly, taught me how I can be both a leader and a team player. Learning and performing dance for seven years has allowed me to hone the ability to complete strenuous tasks while working on improving my skills.

I understand that studying medicine requires dedication, motivation and a prolonged path of learning, which I realise is not easy. However, I believe my personal attributes, determination and the experiences I have encountered can make me a successful medical student.

Personal statement: Example 2 (character count: 3,934)

While undertaking a placement in the First Faculty of Medicine, Charles University, Prague, I learnt how to scrub up. In theatre I observed a temporomandibular joint dysfunction replacement surgery. It was like watching a perfectly put together performance, the protagonists being the multidisciplinary team, and every movement was intricate; the level of focus was patent. There was authentic excitement, I was immersed into the event, I felt a certain empathy with the patient and marvelled at every other character involved in this one story. The experience informed me not only of the complexities involved in surgery but also the sheer level of co-ordinated teamwork.

I was able to notice some obvious contrasts between this experience and one of my previous placements in an emergency medical clinic in rural India. With only one doctor in the whole clinic, long hours were necessary and I found it difficult to fathom how he managed without a more integrated team. From this, I was able to gain an insight into the application of medicine in rural and urban areas. On my final day, an elderly person collapsed in the waiting room. The limited resources did not allow for this patient to be dealt with in an efficient manner. The diagnosis of ventricular tachycardia allowed me to make direct links to my A level Biology content in which the study of the heart and its natural pacemakers are a prominent topic in terms of an organism's response to changes in an environment.

Wanting to study medicine is not something that was an easy decision. My experiences have shown that studying medicine is for someone willing to sacrifice aspects of life that other professions would not have to, but be willing to do so because of a passion and a will to work with people and understand humans, whether anatomically or emotionally.

I have learned valuable lessons from volunteering on a weekly basis at an NHS rehabilitation hospital. A desire to care for patients has been instigated in me as I was fortunate enough to be part of multiple journeys of growth to recovery. I further came to realise this while volunteering in a care home over a period of a year, where I built close relationships with residents and was introduced to geriatrics.

Spending some of my free time in a hospital environment has allowed me to witness the stressful nature of the job: the team operates with the expertise and input of doctors, nurses, physios, the occupational therapist and ward clerks. Having been Head Girl at my previous school, I reflected on my own leadership and teamwork experiences to identify the skillsets that I have developed that will prove valuable being carried forward into medicine. I hope to refine these as part of a medical team.

I have taken my passion of science to places outside of the classroom. This past year I have taken great interest in reading about specific facets of neurology, especially the effect of classical music on the brain. Playing a classical instrument to a high standard myself, including teaching students, phenomena such as the 'Mozart effect' struck me as engaging topics to read and write articles on; one that I particularly enjoyed was the J.S. Jenkins article in which he made alluring links between epilepsy and Mozart.

My understanding of human nature has been supplemented by my love for theatre. Usually science and drama exist in parallel. Being a member of the national youth theatre I have performed in various places across the country and adore the feeling of being part of such a tight-knit group, it's allowed me to develop an invaluable confidence.

Medicine is both a science and an art: it will allow me to fulfil my passion for both. It presents itself as a rich career that is all about life-long learning and continual development.

Personal statement: Example 3 (character count: 3,647)

There is no greater calling than the ability to preserve human life. I have a passion for learning and practising medicine. My interest developed when I visited India as a child. I was struck by the inequality in access to basic health services. I witnessed children suffering because their parents could not afford rudimentary medical treatment. I developed an ambition to work as a doctor in the NHS – to relieve suffering by providing free treatment at the point of use.

I gained insight from a two-week placement at Queen Elizabeth Hospital, Birmingham. I saw treatment and palliative care for numerous conditions, including cancer. I was particularly moved when a scan revealed a tumour in a mother. The neuroradiologist quickly diagnosed it was benign by talking to colleagues. This collegiate approach avoided delay, thereby alleviating the patient's emotional trauma. This taught me that medicine involved teamwork, managing time and emotions, as well as having academic-based skill. I was fascinated by the technology deployed in thrombectomy surgery. I witnessed the removal of a blood clot using fluoroscopy. Seeing mechanical aids used at the cutting edge of medicine illustrated to me that technology was crucial to medical advancement. I learnt that mechanical engineering could be as invaluable to medicine as biology.

During a one-week placement at a GP surgery I gained insight into doctors' every day work and their skills in communicating with patients. I saw doctors advise patients to make lifestyle changes (eg losing weight, reducing cholesterol, exercising more) to avoid illness. This holistic approach taught me that a doctor's role was not just to have skills and knowledge, but also to exercise judgement and communicate diplomatically to persuade patients that prevention is better than cure.

Volunteering at a care home developed my interpersonal skills. Some residents suffered Alzheimer's; I learnt to lower and slow my speech when talking to them, so they could comprehend me. Even menial tasks facilitated conversations with residents, enabling me to develop my confidence and relationships. As part of NCS, we worked with Help for Heroes to enhance our awareness of mental ill health induced by PTSD.

Reading *Surgery Under the Knife*, which gives a historical account of surgery, has taught me how surgical techniques develop and how I will need to keep apprised of new procedures. Reading *When Medicine Went Mad* has taught me the importance of medical ethics to avoid doctors using their training to inflict harm in breach of their Hippocratic Oath. Studying A-level Economics has developed my writing and critical analysis skills, which are invaluable for medical research.

During a mini pupillage with a barrister, I analysed how medical knowledge could be applied outside a clinical setting. The barrister represented a tetraplegic client. I helped the barrister research suitable mechanical aids for her client. My research revealed an array of equipment, often developed for paralympians and injured soldiers. Such science combines physics and biology and represents one of the new frontiers in medical science.

Undertaking military exercises as a Royal Marine Cadet has enhanced my leadership skills, decision making and strategic thinking. I have learnt core field survival skills. I am a qualified children's rugby coach. This training included First Aid. I know how to apply CPR, treat wounds/ hypothermia and how to use a defibrillator. Coaching has aided my critical thinking, communication and authority skills. I have represented my school in rugby, rowing, cricket and hockey. These sports demonstrate my dedication to physical fitness. Academically, I have achieved school attainment awards in biology, chemistry and physics.

A career in medicine will enable me to provide aid to vulnerable people on the most important aspect of their life – their mental and physical health and well-being.

Personal statement: Example 4 (character count: 3,960)

My path into applying for medicine has been slightly unusual. I discovered that I wanted to study medicine while in my first year of an English Literature and French degree; I was enjoying my studies, but felt that something was missing. While working as a Notes Summariser at a GP practice, I found myself fascinated by the stories that patient records held and the impact of medical care on an individual's life. I wondered how it would feel to be involved in offering that care, and realised something missing from my future plans was the meaning that my life could offer to others. I found myself wanting to be in the position of the doctor, so that I could learn more about the world of medicine and help people similar to the individuals I was reading about. I decided, having successfully completed my first year at university, to leave and focus on my ambition of reading medicine, by studying A level Biology and Chemistry. This increased my desire to develop an understanding of medicine's scientific basis, while allowing me to improve my independent study skills which I had developed at university.

As I had already experienced Primary Care, I wanted to understand more about hospital medicine, and so arranged some work experience where I was given the opportunity to shadow a range of medical professionals. I was struck by the teamwork involved, with many different roles working together for the patient to make a successful healthcare service. I found shadowing in oncology thought-provoking, and I felt that the holistic nature of care was particularly important. In cardiology, I witnessed an encounter between a Registrar and an unhappy patient who wanted to go home, and noticed how by allowing them to express how they were feeling, comforting them, and then explaining clearly why they needed to remain in hospital, the situation was successfully resolved. I was able to observe a complicated operation to remove a tumour from the rectum of a patient, which highlighted the technical skill and scientific knowledge required. This was reinforced when I observed a stent being inserted into an artery to prevent a heart attack. It was such a quick operation, but talking to the surgeon afterwards, his comment that it could also be very quick to kill someone through the operation and the responsibility associated with that, has stayed with me.

Working as a Domiciliary Care Worker has given me the skills to manage the care of individuals on my own, and shown me the importance of companionship to those who are elderly or frail. Looking after people with dementia has taught me how to remain patient and clear when communicating.

My neighbour has, very sadly, been diagnosed with MND. Helping to care for her, I have seen first-hand the progression of her disease and her emotional struggle with loss of independence. This experience has shown me the limitations of modern medicine, and taught me the importance of accepting human mortality.

As a youth support leader with St John Ambulance, I helped to organise and deliver Cadet sessions which improved my leadership and teamwork skills. This built on skills that I had gained during my work as a Residential Counsellor with LINES Language Summer School, where I learnt how to relate to individuals from different cultures. Helping young people who were often feeling homesick taught me how acting with empathy and understanding helps make the best of any situation. It interested me to read a *BMJ* article saying that empathy is vital to being a good doctor, but overexposure to pain and suffering can cause empathy to decrease. I feel that it is not always easy to learn from difficult and painful situations, however it is essential to share and reflect on our experiences of suffering so we can improve our empathy.

I have played the piano for 15 years, and have successfully taken my grade 5 and practical musicianship. I now play for relaxation and enjoy the challenge of learning new pieces.

WARNING!

Do not write any of the above passages in your personal statement, as admissions tutors are all too aware of the existence of this book. They also use plagiarism software to determine similarities between scripts. Ensure that your personal statement is not only personal to you, but also honest.

'All I really want to see is a student has a determination to succeed and one who has researched everything about the career path they are looking to undertake. Evidence is king, to misquote another saying. Remember that the person reading the personal statement has read hundreds, in some cases thousands of them before and therefore will be able to distinguish between what is real and what is embellished. Keep it interesting but above all else, keep it personal. Be truthful to why you want to study the course and what you have done about researching that. Remember the value of work experience is to educate and inform and confirm to you that this path is the one you want to take. Oh and don't swallow a thesaurus! Understand each word you write. Communication is the hallmark of a good doctor.'

Advice from an admissions tutor

6 | The interview process

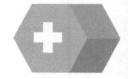

Once you've submitted your UCAS application, you must wait to hear from each of the universities you have applied to. If you meet their entry criteria and they feel that your application is strong in the areas they deem to be most important, they may call you for interview. The universities use interviews to find out first hand whether the picture painted by your application is accurate and to investigate whether you have the skills necessary to succeed on the course.

Interviews for medical school usually take place between December and March each application cycle. While the thought of attending an interview can be somewhat scary, with careful preparation and practice it can ultimately turn out to be a rewarding experience.

At the time of writing, Covid-19 is presenting a big challenge to universities in terms of organising interviews. It is expected that all universities in the 2020–21 application cycle will hold online interviews, although it won't be clear for a number of months what is likely to happen in the 2021–22 cycle. Regardless of whether an interview occurs online or in person, the general principles remain the same, and so there is no difference in the preparation that needs to be carried out.

In this section, we will consider both multiple mini interviews (MMIs) and panel interviews, and the specific steps you will need to go through in order to prepare yourself, as well as more general interview pointers. Most of this guidance will be relevant to both types of interview and give appropriate general interview advice, but differences will be highlighted where necessary.

Making your interview a success

If you are invited to an interview, you need to prepare thoroughly for it, as you will not be given a second chance if you do not perform well. As with most other activities, the more you prepare and practise, the better your chance of success. Interviews can be stressful and you will be nervous, and so practice interviews are an important part of your preparation.

In this chapter, we look at common types of interview question and provide you with suggestions about how to approach them. You can then practise using the list of sample interview questions.

The questions that we look at in this chapter have all been asked at medical school interviews over recent years, and have been provided by students who have been interviewed and by members of medical school interview panels. You cannot always prepare for the odd, unpredictable questions that are bound to crop up, but the interviewers are not trying to catch you out, and they can be relied on to ask questions based on most of the general themes that are discussed here.

For most questions, there is not a single 'correct' answer, and, even if there were, you shouldn't try to memorise them and repeat them as you would lines in a theatre script. The purpose of presenting these questions, and some strategies for answering them, is to help you think about your answers before the interview and to enable you to put forward your own views clearly and with confidence.

When you have read through this section, and thought about the questions, arrange for someone to sit down with you and take you through the mock interview questions. (You might find it helpful to record the interview for later analysis.) You might be interested in the views of medical professionals on the qualities that they look for. These views will not have changed; in fact, time and time again they are emphasised by professionals in this field.

> 'The medical schools are looking for well-rounded individuals that have interests in lots of different things, should be personable in order to be good with patients and have a good scientific knowledge which is par for the programme really. They are looking for lifelong learners, with a holistic approach to patients and able to maintain a good work-life balance. At times it can be a tough job and at times a very rewarding job and so they want people who can balance those stresses.'
>
> Dr Vicki Cooney, GP and Medical Interviewer,
> Hammersmith and Fulham

> 'The innate characteristics of a good doctor are beneficence and the capacity to engage with the knowledge necessary for informed practice.'
>
> Dr Allan Cumming, Associate Dean of Teaching,
> University of Edinburgh

> 'I think that you are born with some personal qualities, such as the ability to get on with people, to empathise with their distress, to inspire confidence in others, and to carry anxiety. Such qualities are very difficult to train into a person. A good doctor also needs knowledge and the experience of implementing that knowledge.'
>
> Mike Shooter,
> President of the Royal College of Psychiatrists

'Medicine should always be regarded as a life commitment and not just a job. The demands put on you as a medical student and as a doctor will far exceed that of a standard job that some of your peers are able to land after just a few years of study and experience. It follows that making a commitment of this kind should not be taken lightly, especially when we see the strains and pressures put on the NHS and doctors which will ultimately lead to compromising patient care and safety. No one wants to be treated by an average doctor, in the same way as we would not want to be in a plane flown by an average pilot! So expect to be expected to be super human even when you know you aren't.

'In other countries, such as the US, medical school is something you apply for after you have spent several years studying a degree or pre-med – I think this is a much wiser career choice as it will give you a few years to not only mature academically but to also establish your true calling. Studying medicine as a graduate may add on a few more years of study before you become a doctor, but it actually enhances your chances of getting the medical job you want – a reason so many medical students choose to intercalate. A doctor represents trust, integrity, compassion and someone who can make a significant difference to someone's life in an instant. Once you have honestly convinced yourself that you have indeed got what it takes, convincing admissions officers will be so much easier – learn to enjoy the pressure and remember that becoming a great doctor is a journey and not a target, so take your time.'

Kal Makwana, Executive Chairman of Medipathways

Typical interview themes and how to handle them (for both panel and MMI)

Although some of these questions will come up directly in some interviews, you may not be asked all of them explicitly. In spite of this, it is still worth considering and preparing responses to them as they will provide a solid foundation of ideas that you can use for questions that pick up on similar themes.

1. Why do you want to become a doctor?

This is the question that is most likely to come up in one form or another and, as such, tends to be the most over-rehearsed one by applicants. There are no correct and incorrect answers to this question, but some areas to avoid include the following.

- My father is a doctor and I want to be like him.
- The money's good and unemployment among doctors is low.
- The careers teacher told me to apply.
- It's glamorous.
- I want to join a respected profession, so it is either this or law.

Try answering the question now. Most sixth-formers find it quite hard to respond and are often not sure why they want to be a doctor. The interviewers will be sympathetic, but they do require an answer that sounds convincing. If you are struggling with this question, consider some of the approaches suggested below.

The story (option A)
You tell the interesting (and true) story of how you have always been interested in medicine, how you have made an effort to find out what is involved by visiting your local hospital, working with your GP, etc. and how this long-term and deep-seated interest has now become something of a passion. With this option, be prepared to back up your general statements with experiences from your placements.

The story (option B)
You tell the interesting (and true) story of how you, or a close relative, suffered from an illness that brought you into contact with the medical profession. This experience made you think of becoming a doctor and, since then, you have made an effort to find out what is involved … (as before).

The logical elimination of alternatives (option C)
In this approach you have analysed your career options and decided that you want to spend your life in a scientific environment (you have enjoyed science at school) but would find pure research too impersonal. Therefore the idea of a career that combines the excitement of scientific investigation with a great deal of human contact is attractive. Since discovering that medicine offers this combination, you have investigated it (and other alternatives) thoroughly (visits to hospitals, GPs, etc.) and have become passionately committed to your decision.

The problems with this approach are that:

- they will have heard it all before
- you will find it harder to convince them of your passion for medicine as it can seem quite a cold way to choose a career.

Fascination with people (option D)
Some applicants can honestly claim to have a real interest in people and feel that a career in medicine would give them an opportunity to develop this. When coupled with an interest in biology, this can be a compelling argument due to the well-developed people skills that a successful doctor must have.

Answer with conviction

Your answer must be well considered and convincing, sound natural and not be over-rehearsed. Although an interview is a formal process, the more relaxed and natural your tone is, the better your chances are of success. Bear in mind that most of your interviewers will be doctors, and they (hopefully) will have chosen medicine because they, like you, had a burning desire to do so. Statements (as long as they are supported by evidence of practical research) such as 'and the more work I did at St James's, the more I realised that medicine is what I desperately want to do' are quite acceptable and far more convincing than saying 'medicine is the only career that combines science and the chance to work with people', because it isn't!

> 'The candidates who do best are those who are able to find something to be a good stress relief for them as the course can be quite overwhelming, from the interview process through to the job. We are looking for students who can balance their time so they do not burn out. In terms of an application, they need to be a reflective learner and to work out what kind of doctor they want to be, as this will affect the way they approach the degree. There is no substitute to life experience, and we are looking for candidates who can bring themselves to both the interview and the job. Be confident and assured when you are at the interview; we are friendly and just want to get the best out of you, not make you so nervous you cannot even answer the questions. Try and enjoy the experience.'
>
> *Advice from an admissions tutor*

2. What have you done to show your commitment to medicine and to the community?

This should tie in with your UCAS application. Your answer should demonstrate that you have a genuine interest in helping others. Ideally, you will have a track record of regular visits to your local hospital or hospice, where you will have had interactions with patients and staff and seen the less attractive side of patient care (such as cleaning bedpans). Acceptable alternatives are regular visits to an elderly person to do their chores, or volunteering for charities that care for disadvantaged groups. It is important that you can give details of experience that you have had while carrying out these placements in order to show that they are genuine and that you have taken time to reflect on what you have seen.

It isn't sufficient to have worked in a laboratory, out of sight of patients, or to have done so little work as to be trivial: 'I once walked around the ward of the local hospital.' The interviewer may ask: 'If you enjoyed working in the hospital so much, why don't you want to become a nurse?' This is a tough question. You need to indicate that, while you admire enormously the work that nurses do, you would like the challenge of diagnosis and of deciding what treatment should be given.

You also need to ask yourself why admissions tutors ask about work experience. It is not a tick-box exercise, rather they want to know whether you were there in body only, or if you were genuinely engaged with what was happening around you.

3. Why have you applied to this medical school?

Areas to avoid are:

- it has a good reputation (all UK medical schools do)
- you have low entrance requirements
- my father studied here
- it is close to the city's nightclubs.

Some of the reasons that you might have are given below.

- **Talking to people.** You have made a thorough investigation of a number of the medical schools that you have considered, by talking to your teachers, doctors and medical students you encountered during your work experience, and current students. They have given you a good picture of what it would be like to study here and have all said that university, course and style of teaching would suit you perfectly.
- **The course.** You have read the course details and feel that it is structured in a way that suits your style of study and medical interests. You like the fact that it is integrated/traditional/PBL/CBL and that students are brought into contact with patients at an early stage. Another related reason might be that you are attracted by the subject-based or systems-based teaching approach.
- **The open day.** You visited a number of medical schools' open days (either in person or virtually) and this one was by far the most interesting and informative. While attending, you talked to current medical students. You have spoken to the admissions tutor about your particular situation and asked their advice about suitable work experience, and he or she was particularly encouraging and helpful. You feel that the general atmosphere is one you would love to be part of.
- **The town/city/area.** Although you want to avoid discussing the nightlife or social scene, it is perfectly acceptable to talk about aspects of the local area that appeal to you.

'Treat the additional questionnaire and any written correspondence as though they have the same importance as the exams and the aptitude tests. Any time the university asks for information, it is because they are seriously considering your application and therefore any half-hearted efforts will not be viewed favourably by the department. Simply call it good practice in diligence for the profession.'

Advice from an admissions tutor

4. Questions designed to assess your knowledge of the world of medicine

No one expects you to know all about your future career before you start at medical school, but they do expect you to have made an effort to find out something about it. If you are really interested in medicine, you will have a reasonable idea of common illnesses and diseases, and you will be aware of topical issues through your wider reading and research. The questions aimed at testing your knowledge of medicine can be broadly divided into six areas:

i.   major medical issues
ii.   the medical profession
iii. the National Health Service and funding health
iv.   private medicine
v.   ethical questions
vi.   other issues.

'The purpose of the interview is not to intimidate you, it is to get you to tell us why this is what you want above all else and what you have learnt. If we invite you to interview, you need to remember that it is because you have already jumped over a number of hurdles where many will have stumbled, and you are being seriously considered for a place at the medical school. This should give you a certain amount of confidence and hopefully allow you to enjoy the experience. Remember to maintain eye contact and body language throughout the interview, if you don't know the answer you can ask for clarification; however, try to give it a go; we will re-direct your answer if we need to and, most importantly, stick to what you know and not what you have *not* done please. We enjoy the interview process as meeting so many candidates from different backgrounds is the best part of this job. If you have any questions in advance, do not hesitate to contact the Admissions department – we can be friendly, despite the myth.'

Advice from an admissions tutor

i. Major medical issues

The interviewers will expect you to be interested in medicine and to have a general awareness of current issues and new treatments. The best way to develop your understanding of this is to regularly read news articles and keep a file of the ones of interest to you and take the time to reflect on and record the illnesses and treatments that you came across during your work experience placements.

Keep a file of cuttings

Make sure that you read *New Scientist*, *Student BMJ* and, on a daily basis, a high-quality newspaper, news website or news app, that has a health or medical section. The *Independent* has excellent coverage of current health issues, and the *Guardian*'s health section is interesting and informative. Newspapers' websites often group articles thematically, which can save time. Taking as little as five minutes each day to read the most topical health news will ultimately have a major impact on developing your understanding.

Topical illnesses

At any one time, the media tend to concentrate on one or two topical diseases which dominate coverage for a short period before fading into the background. Over the last 30 years, Ebola, CJD, SARS, bird flu, swine flu and Zika among others, resulted in relatively small numbers of deaths, even though they dominated the news at the time. At present, Covid-19 dominates the news headlines, due to the widespread and deadly impact it has had on the global population. As there has been so much media coverage of Covid-19, there will be no excuse for not having a solid understanding of the virus, its effects and its legacy across the globe.

While some of these diseases may not have a significant and lasting impact, they are often interesting in scientific terms, and the fact that they have been discussed in the media makes it likely that they will come up at interview. The next few paragraphs discuss some examples of diseases and illnesses that have been brought into the public eye and so it is worth having a good general knowledge of them.

Covid-19, also known as Coronavirus, is an infectious viral disease that spreads mainly via droplets of saliva expelled by coughing or sneezing. The virus causes a range of symptoms, which may include a high temperature, a persistent cough and a change in smell or taste. The majority of people who contract the virus experience only mild symptoms and recover quickly. However, some individuals, including older people and those with underlying medical conditions, are more susceptible to developing serious complications.

At the time of writing, there have been over 91 million recorded cases of COVID-19 globally, with nearly 2 million deaths. It is likely that the official number of infections is a massive underestimate due to individuals with mild symptoms not being tested.

The search for effective treatments and vaccines for Covid-19 provides a useful insight into the discovery, development and testing of drugs. Particularly interesting has been the global race to discover safe and effective vaccines. The various different approaches to this are well worth researching as they link to a number of topics on the A level Biology specification.

Mental health conditions, including depression, anxiety and bipolar disorders are a major group of illnesses among all age groups. Over the past decade, there have been concerted efforts to raise awareness of these conditions and, as such, there is significant and ongoing media coverage. Treatments for mental health conditions can include lifestyle changes, therapy and medication.

Lyme disease is an infection that can be caused by a tick bite. The disease has a variety of symptoms, affecting the skin, heart, joints and nervous system. It is also known as borrelia or borreliosis. The disease is caused by the *Borrelia burgdorferi* microorganism, which is present on ticks that live on deer. The symptoms of the disease, which first manifests itself as a red spot caused by the tick bite, include headaches, muscle pain and swollen lymph glands, and eventually the nervous system is affected. The symptoms may be apparent days after the tick bite, but in some cases they only present themselves months or even years later.

These diseases and illnesses have become more well known in recent times and, as a result, have gained more media coverage. This has had the effect of causing greater concern to the general public, who may have been unaware of their existence otherwise.

The big killers

Heart disease, cancer and stroke are the main causes of death in the UK. Make sure you know the factors that contribute to them and the strategies for prevention and treatment. You can read more about this in Chapter 7.

The global picture

You may well be asked about what is happening on a global scale. You should know about the biggest killers (infectious diseases and circulatory diseases), trends in population changes, the role of the World Health Organization (WHO), and the differences in medical treatments between developed and developing countries. You can read more about this in Chapter 7.

The Human Genome Project and gene therapy

You would be wise to familiarise yourself with developments in the field of genetic research, starting with the discovery of the double helix structure of DNA by Crick and Watson in 1953. You should find out all that you can about:

- recombinant DNA technology (gene therapy, genetic engineering)
- genetic screening
- personalised medicine based on your genome
- cloning
- stem cell research
- GM crops
- genetic enhancement of livestock
- genetic engineering of organisms to produce pharmaceutical products.

Diet, exercise and the environment

The maintenance of health on a national scale isn't simply a matter of waiting until people get ill and then rushing in with surgery or medicine to cure them. Many diseases can be prevented by a healthy diet, not smoking, taking exercise and living in a healthy environment.

In this context, a healthy environment means one where food and water are uncontaminated by bacteria and living quarters are well ventilated, warm and dry. The huge advance in health and life expectancy since the middle of the nineteenth century owes much more to these factors than to the achievements of modern medicine.

However, with unhealthy eating habits and a sedentary lifestyle becoming more prevalent, one of the biggest problems developing in the UK today is obesity. It is an ever-increasing issue and treating the associated problems costs the NHS more and more money each year. For more information on this, see Chapter 7.

> **TIP!**
>
> When discussing medical topics, try to use the correct terminology. However, if you are discussing a topic, do not be put off if you are not sure of the exact technical terms. It is better to show that you have a general grasp of an issue, even if it is not to the highest level of understanding.

ii. The medical profession

Although having a well-developed knowledge of health and disease is important, it is also vital to have an understanding of the medical profession and what being a doctor entails.

Questions in this area tend to relate to your understanding of the skills and attributes that a doctor needs. Good starting points for developing your understanding of the career are the BMA website, which has extensive guidance (www.bma.org.uk/advice/career/studying-medicine), and the GMC website, which has the 'Outcomes for Graduates' document, sometimes known as 'Tomorrow's Doctors' (www.gmc-uk.org/education/standards-guidance-and-curricula/standards-and-outcomes/outcomes-for-graduates).

Begin by considering the importance of the technical skills that a doctor needs: the ability to carry out a thorough examination, to diagnose accurately and quickly what is wrong, and the skill to choose and organise the correct treatment and the precision to carry out treatment.

After this comes the ability to communicate effectively and sympathetically with the patient so that he or she can understand and participate in the treatment. The most important part of communication is listening.

Communication skills also have an important role to play in treatment – studies have shown that some patients get better more quickly when they feel involved and part of the medical team.

Other important skills include organisation, teamwork, empathy and working under pressure.

For each of these skills and the others that you identify, it is vital that you are prepared to discuss experiences from your life that illustrate that you have the skill or have taken steps to develop that skill. For example, you might say 'I was able to demonstrate my ability to work as part of a team during my Duke of Edinburgh expedition when I ...'

Also make sure that you can define each skill. A good example of this is from an interview at Brighton and Sussex Medical School, where a student was asked to explain what empathy was and to distinguish it from sympathy.

iii. The National Health Service and funding health

With issues relating to the NHS dominating so much of the news, it is vital that you have a clear picture of the issues it faces. This will allow you to deal with any questions or scenarios that arise in relation to this in an interview.

An application to a medical school is also an application for a job, and you should have taken the trouble to find out something about your likely future employer. You should be aware of the structure of the NHS and the role that clinical commissioning groups and foundation trusts play. You need to know about the way in which doctors are trained, and the career paths that are open to medical graduates. When you are doing your work experience, you should take every opportunity to discuss the problems in the NHS with the doctors whom you meet. They will be able to give you first-hand accounts of what is happening, and this is an effective way of identifying the big issues that you can then go on to research further.

The key issues currently surrounding the NHS that should be investigated further are:

- the impact of Covid-19 on the provision of NHS services
- the impact of Covid-19 on NHS staff
- funding (or lack thereof)
- staff shortages
- the social care crisis
- the cost of treating problems related to lifestyle diseases such as obesity
- caring for an ageing population
- steps being taken towards privatisation.

iv. Private medicine

Another area that needs careful thought concerns private medicine. Don't forget that many consultants have flourishing private practices and rely on private work for a major part of their income.

Most people agree that if you are run over by a bus you should be taken to hospital and treated at the taxpayers' expense. In general, urgent treatment for serious and life-threatening conditions should be provided by the NHS and we should all contribute towards its cost. On the other hand, most of us would agree that someone who wants to change the shape of their nose with cosmetic surgery should pay for the operation themselves.

Having established these two extremes, one is left to argue about the point where the two systems meet. Should there be a firm dividing line between where both the NHS and private medicine operate? A good example of this is related to the provision of surgery for joint replacement. Most hip replacement operations are not a matter of life-or-death so should they be provided on the NHS, even if there is massive demand for them due to the ageing population of the UK? Or should they only be provided privately due to the limited resources of the NHS? Currently, there are strict criteria for referrals for this surgery and very long waiting lists, which effectively mean that this treatment is rationed.

You could also point out that private medicine does not necessarily harm the NHS. For example, the NHS has a problem of waiting lists. If 10 people are standing in a queue for a bus, everyone benefits if four of those waiting jump into a taxi – providing, of course, that they don't persuade the bus driver to drive it!

v. Ethical questions

Medical ethics is a fascinating area of moral philosophy. You won't be expected to answer questions on the finer points of philosophy, but many questions, scenarios and role plays in interviews will have their basis in medical ethics.

A patient who refuses treatment

You could be presented with a scenario, and asked what you would do in the situation. For example, you have to inform a patient that he has cancer. Without radiotherapy and chemotherapy his life expectancy is likely to be a matter of months. The patient tells you that he or she does not wish to be treated. What would you do if you were in this situation? The first thing to remember is that the interviewer is not asking you this question because he or she wants to know what the answer to this problem is. Questions of this nature are designed to see whether you can look at problems from different angles, weigh up arguments, use your knowledge of medical issues to come to a conclusion, and produce coherent and structured answers.

A good technique for answering 'What would you do if you were a doctor and ...' questions is to start by discussing the information that you would need, or the questions that you might ask the patient. In the above example, you would ask these questions.

- How old is the patient?
- Does the patient have any other medical conditions that might affect his or her life expectancy?
- Why is the patient refusing the treatment?

The answer to these questions would then determine what you would do next. The patient could be refusing treatment for religious or moral reasons; it might simply be that he or she has heard stories about the side-effects of the treatment you have recommended. One possible route would be to give him or her contact details of a suitable support group, counselling service or information centre.

A classic case is someone who refuses a life-saving blood transfusion because it contravenes his or her religious beliefs. You may feel that this is acceptable for the individual in question, but what if, on these grounds, a parent refuses to allow a baby's life to be saved by a transfusion? Similarly, in a well-publicised legal case, a woman refused to allow a caesarean delivery of her baby. The judge ruled that the wishes of the mother could be overruled. It is worth noting that the NHS (as a representative of the state) has no right to keep a patient in hospital against his or her will unless the medical team and relatives use the powers of the Mental Health Act.

The BMA website has excellent resources to help you navigate your way through ethical scenarios and reading and digesting these is a great place to start your preparation. The Ethics toolkit can be found at www. bma.org.uk/advice-and-support/ethics. Take the time to look at and understand each of the sections as they can be directly used to inform your response to any scenario. It is impossible that one scenario will relate to all areas of medical ethics, so it is important that you identify the areas that are best suited and discuss these in context.

Euthanasia

To answer questions on euthanasia, start by making sure that you know the following correct terminology, and the law.

- **Suicide.** The act of killing oneself intentionally.
- **Physician-assisted suicide.** This involves a doctor intentionally giving a person advice on or the means to commit suicide although they are not directly involved in administering those means.
- **Euthanasia.** Euthanasia is a deliberate act or omission whose primary intention is to end another's life. Literally, it means a gentle or easy death, but it has come to signify a deliberate intervention with the intention to kill someone, often described as the 'mercy killing' of people in pain with terminal illnesses.
    - **Voluntary euthanasia** – when a person voluntarily asks for help to end their life.
    - **Non-voluntary euthanasia** – when a person cannot give consent and as a result a decision is made on their behalf, possibly because they had previously made their wishes known about their life ending.
- **Double effect.** The principle of double effect provides the justification for the provision of medical treatment that has a negative effect, although the intention is to provide an overall positive effect. The principle permits an act that foreseeably has both good and bad effects, provided that the good effect is the reason for acting and is not caused by the bad. A common example is the provision of essential pain-relieving drugs in terminal care, at the risk of shortening life. Pain relief is the intention and outweighs the risk of shortening life.
- **Non-treatment.** Competent adults have the right to refuse any treatment, including life-prolonging procedures. The British Medical Association (BMA) does not consider valid treatment refusal by a patient to be suicide. Respecting a competent, informed patient's treatment refusal is not assisting suicide.
- **Withdrawing/withholding life-prolonging medical treatment.** Not all treatment with the potential to prolong life has to be provided in all circumstances, especially if its effect is seen as extending the dying process. Cardio-pulmonary resuscitation of a terminally ill cancer patient is an extreme example. In deciding which treatment should be offered, the expectation must be that the advantages outweigh the drawbacks for the individual patient.

Currently in the UK the act of intentionally killing an individual, even if carried out as a mercy-killing, is considered to be manslaughter or murder, depending on the circumstances. This carries the maximum of a life sentence. Assisted suicide remains a crime in the UK, punishable by up to 14 years in prison. This is a very contentious issue and, as you can imagine, even within the medical community opinion is divided. In short, it questions the ethical conundrum of the right of the individual to 'die with dignity' when they so wish versus the argument that it goes against moral and religious teaching and that it is against God's law to take a life. The nature of this ethical dilemma is central to the role of a doctor, as some would argue further that it also goes against the moral duty of a doctor, which is to prolong life instead of shortening it.

In September 2015, MPs were allowed a free vote to debate changing the law towards assisted dying in the House of Commons, concluding three to one against giving a second reading to a Bill to change the law. While not a legal case, in 2015 Simon Binner made the headlines as he posted on his LinkedIn page details of his impending date of death and funeral, trying, in doing so, to bring the issue to the public consciousness again – to say that everyone has a choice.

As this is a controversial question, it is one that is often used in interviews. What must be remembered is that aside from your own beliefs, whether you do or don't support euthanasia, the de facto position in the UK is that assisted suicides are currently illegal. You need to make it clear that you understand this before expressing any further ideas or opinions. To date, Swiss-based group, Dignitas, has helped over 450 UK citizens to commit suicide. Dignitas was founded in 1998 to help people with chronic diseases to die, honouring the wishes of the patient and those around them to end their suffering. There is currently nothing stopping UK nationals from travelling to Switzerland and being assisted to commit suicide, but, as the law stands, loved ones and friends may be prosecuted if they help. See Chapter 7 for more information.

One possible question is: 'Could you withdraw treatment from a patient for whom the prognosis was very poor, who seemed to enjoy no quality of life and who was in great pain?' The answer to this question must recognise that a decision like this could not be taken without the benefit of full medical training and some experience, together with the advice of colleagues and the fullest consultation with the patient and his or her relations, as well as knowing your position according to the law. If, after that process, it was clear that life support should be withdrawn, then, and only then, would you take your decision.

vi. Other issues
'Should smokers be treated on the NHS?'

On the one hand, it is certainly true that smoking is a contributory factor in heart disease. Is it fair to expect the community as a whole to spend a great deal of money on, for example, coronary artery bypass surgery if the patient refuses to abandon behaviour that could jeopardise the long-term effectiveness of the operation? Conversely, one can argue that all citizens and certainly all taxpayers have the right to treatment, irrespective of their lifestyle choices. Further to this, one can argue that taxes paid on cigarettes add up to more than the cost of treatment.

'Is it right to ration healthcare?'

Suppose you have resources for one operation but two critically ill patients – how do you decide which one to save? Could you, for example, choose between someone who is morbidly obese and someone who had a heart attack while running a marathon? Or suppose that you can perform six hip replacement operations for the cost of one coronary artery bypass. Heart bypass operations save lives; hip replacements merely improve life. Which option should you go for?

Events are constantly bringing fresh moral issues associated with medicine into the public arena. It is important that you read the papers and maintain an awareness of the current 'hot' issues.

5. Questions aimed at finding out whether you have the necessary skills to be a doctor

One of the reasons for interviewing you is to see whether you will fit successfully into both the medical school and the medical profession. The interviewers will try to find out if your views and approach to life are likely to make you an acceptable colleague in a profession that, to a great extent, depends on teamwork. This does not mean that they want to hear views identical to their own. On the contrary, they will welcome ideas that are refreshing and interesting. What they do not like to hear is arrogance, lies, bigotry or tabloid headlines.

The vast majority of questions, regardless of what they are about, will have another important purpose: to assess your ability to communicate in a friendly and effective way with strangers even when under pressure. This skill will be very important when you come to deal with patients.

You may be asked to explain or to act out in a role play how you would deal with a minor accident, for example. You are reversing out of your driveway when you accidentally run over your neighbour's cat, although nobody else has seen you do it. You have to break the news to your neighbour. What do you do?

The interviewer is looking for evidence of the following:

- you clearly communicate the events to your neighbour
- you show a caring and empathetic attitude
- you are able to successfully deal with a person who is upset or angry.

6. Questions about your UCAS application

The personal statement section, in which you write about yourself, is a fertile area for interviewers to base questions on. It is therefore vital to keep a copy of your personal statement so you can brush up on what you have written in advance of the interview.

If you have mentioned anything specific in your statement that is of interest to you, make sure that you can discuss it if asked. For example, if you have mentioned that you completed an EPQ based on the incidence and spread of avian flu, you should ensure that you can give an overview of your findings.

This is why it is particularly important to ensure that everything in your statement is truthful; anything that you have exaggerated or been untruthful about could potentially come back to haunt you at this point.

7. Questions about how you might contribute to the life of the medical school

These questions can come in many forms and could either focus on how you have contributed to your school or college in the past or how you intend to contribute to university life in the future.

The best approach is to give an answer that demonstrates that you understand the balance needed between study and extracurricular pursuits. However, this type of question is not usually designed to catch you out; it is often a genuine enquiry about whether you have a life beyond your studies and can relax as well as work hard.

You may find it helpful to know that, in one London medical school, the interviewers are told to ask themselves if the candidate has made good use of the opportunities available to them, and whether they have the personal qualities and interests appropriate to student life and a subsequent career in medicine. A lack of evidence of participation in life beyond the curriculum is unlikely to be a positive factor.

8. Unpredictable questions

Even with all of the preparation in the world, there is no way that every question or topic can be pre-empted. If you get asked a question that you have never considered before, try to think about the skills that they are trying to test. This can often help you to demystify the random scenario that you have been given. Often in these scenarios, just being a generally nice, caring and thoughtful human being will help you to give a solid answer, even if you are unsure of the correct approach. Some examples of questions and scenarios are as follows.

- 'If you won £20 million on the lottery, what would you do with it?'
- 'Tell me about your family.'

- 'You start discussing a medical issue with a patient, but they are more concerned about telling you about their washing machine that is broken. How do you deal with the situation?'

In each of these situations, make sure you stay calm and don't panic. If you panic, you are more likely to rush your answer and say something you don't mean. If the question has really surprised you, take a few seconds to plan the key ideas that you wish to discuss rather than just rushing straight into something. However, you still need to treat these questions as seriously as ones that are directly connected to medicine. Also make sure that you don't take offence at the fact that the interviewer is deviating from what you think should be happening in a medical interview; one student got quite aggressive in an interview because she thought she wasn't being asked the questions that she was expecting. Avoid this at all costs!

Although some degree of openness and honesty are useful for these sort of questions, make sure you avoid saying anything that is going to leave a negative impression. For example, telling the interviewer that you hate your family and spend all of your time arguing with them is not going to do anything to impress them, even if it is true!

Another question that interviewees always fear is being asked about something scientific or technical that they have never heard of. For example: 'What is the drug x used for?'

You are not expected to have the knowledge that a qualified doctor has and so you would only be asked this type of question if the drug in question had been in the news recently, or if you had mentioned something related to it in your personal statement. So your pre-interview preparation (making sure you are up to date with recent events and being familiar with your personal statement) will help you here.

This type of question can also be a way to see how you handle yourself in difficult situations and when put under stress. There may be no expectation that you will know about this topic and it might just be to see how your thought processes work or if you can synthesise ideas and information based on your general knowledge and understanding.

Multiple Mini Interviews (MMIs)

In the past, the vast majority of medical interviews have been panel-based, where two or more interviewers ask applicants a series of questions in a similar fashion to a traditional job interview. However, in recent years, the majority of universities have moved towards the system of multiple mini interviews (MMIs).

The MMI is designed to judge the suitability of a candidate to study medicine, and is felt to give a more accurate indication of future academic performance during the course. This style of interview will have some similarities with the panel interview; however, the major difference is that applicants participate in a number of small interviews and tasks rather than just sitting in one place answering questions for the whole interview. For example, the MMI at the University of Birmingham consists of seven six-minute mini interviews. The format of each station will vary, but you will receive instructions explaining what you will be required to do, so ensure that you listen carefully and read any written instructions to give you a good idea of what you will be facing.

There are two main reasons for medical schools using this type of interview. Firstly, research has suggested that traditional panel interviews give a poor indication of the likely performance of the interviewee as an undergraduate; the MMI improves on this. Secondly, one of the major criticisms of the panel interview is that students can be heavily coached on the vast majority of question types and, as a result, do not give an accurate indication of their personality and character attributes. MMIs are therefore specifically designed to test those attributes of the interviewee that are unlikely to be improved by participating in preparation courses. They thereby allow the medical school to build a truer picture of what each candidate is like.

Some universities are relatively tight-lipped about the exact detail of the MMI and give little information to the interviewees, while others are more open to sharing the details of exactly what will be faced. Queen's University Belfast gives detailed exemplar material and short tutorial video clips illustrating what will be faced at each station (visit www.qub. ac.uk/schools/mdbs/Study/Medicine/HowtoApply/MMIs).

The stations are carefully designed to assess attributes such as:

- compassion and empathy
- initiative and resilience
- interpersonal and communication skills
- organisational and problem-solving skills; decision making and critical thinking
- team working
- insight and integrity.

If you will be having an MMI then it would be a good idea to ask multiple members of staff at your school to ask you different questions and get you to think on your feet.

Role plays in MMIs

As stated earlier, the bulk of skills tested in an MMI are similar to those tested in a panel interview. However, one of the biggest differences you will notice about the MMI is the possibility of being asked to 'act out' a scenario in a role play situation These may, but are not guaranteed to, have a medical basis, but will definitely not rely on your knowledge of science or first aid. The point of these stations is therefore to assess attributes such as communication, compassion and calmness under pressure. An example follows.

'You are approached by your elderly neighbour, whose husband has just died. Your neighbour hasn't left her home in three months, but has an upcoming hospital appointment at a hospital that is 20 miles away. She is anxious about attending the hospital appointment and is considering not going. How would you deal with this situation?'

In this situation, you would be expected to start communicating with this person and trying to find out what their worries were, while at the same time reassuring them and trying to keep them calm. You may also think about trying to suggest some solutions to the problems she is facing. Commonly, the person playing the role will be asked to act upset, angry or confused to see how you respond. It is worth trying to practise these with friends or family members in advance to get a feel for how you would react.

Sample MMI questions

Below are some sample MMI questions from recent medical interviews. They are based on broadly the same skills that are tested in a panel interview, although there tends to be more ethical scenario and role play work to do.

- Scenario: 'You are a medical student, and a friend of yours approaches you, telling you that they are feeling anxious and stressed about the upcoming exams.'
  How do you respond to this?
- What would you say are your strengths, giving an example of when you demonstrated each strength.
- What qualities do you have that would make you a good doctor?
- Scenario: 'You are a medical student undertaking a placement at a GP clinic. During an appointment, the doctor is asked to take an emergency phone call. Hence, the doctor asks that you take the patient's blood pressure while he answers the phone call outside. As the doctor leaves the room, the patient begins to show discomfort and unease, and refuses to let you take their blood pressure.'
  How would you respond to the patient?
  What would you do to calm the patient down?
  Why do you think the patient doesn't want you to take their blood pressure?
- How do you know when you are stressed?
- Scenario: 'You are a first-year medical student who is part of a WhatsApp group with a couple of other medical students, one of them being a third-year student called Oscar. Oscar has been

frequently sending pictures of patients without any personal details, and has even been laughing and making fun of their maladies. After a while, you start to think that perhaps this isn't right, so you voice your concerns to the group. Most participants agree not to continue with the activity; however, Oscar says that you shouldn't be so worried and that everyone does it. Thus, he continues to send pictures of patients.'

Why are Oscar's actions wrong?

How would you respond to Oscar?

- Describe a failing of the NHS and explain why it is a problem.
- You are provided with a needle and thread and asked to pick it up with surgical scissors. You then need to use the needle to thread the pattern that is provided using the scissors.

Your questions for the interviewers

In panel interviews you may get the opportunity to ask questions of the people who have interviewed you. Bear in mind that the interviews are carefully timed, and that your attempts to impress the panel with 'clever' questions may do quite the opposite. The golden rule is: only ask a question if you are genuinely interested in the answer (which, of course, you were unable to find during your careful reading of the prospectus and website). Some medical schools will not allow you to ask questions of the interviewing panel and it is extremely unlikely that you will be able to ask questions during an MMI. Questions can be asked of other staff or current students during the time you are there, but not in the interview itself.

Questions to avoid

- What is the structure of the first year of the course?
- Will I be able to live in halls of residence?
- When will I first have contact with patients?
- Can you tell me about the intercalated BSc option?

As well as being dull questions, the answers to these will be available in the prospectus and on the website, and you will show that you have obviously not done any serious research.

One final piece of advice on interviews: keep your answers relatively short and to the point. Nothing is more challenging for an interviewer than dealing with an answer that rambles on. Make sure your answer is detailed, but at the same time, don't be tempted to wander off into areas that don't relate to the question. If your answer does go on too long, expect to be abruptly interrupted; the interviewers aren't trying to be purposefully rude when they do this, but they do have limited time to get through all of the questions.

Mock interview questions

As explained at the beginning of the chapter, interview technique for both types of interview can be improved with practice. You can use this section of the book as a source of mock interview questions. Your interviewer should ask supplementary questions as appropriate. Remember that you won't be asked anywhere near all of these questions, but attempting them will help to sharpen your thought processes and ability to deal with any unexpected questions.

Your motivation to study medicine
- Tell us about yourself.
- Why do you want to be a doctor? What do you want to achieve in medicine?
- What steps have you taken to try to find out whether you really do want to become a doctor? What do you think are the main challenges of becoming a doctor/studying medicine?
- What factors might be behind a student dropping out of medical school?
- How do you deal with stress?

Knowledge of the medical school and teaching methods
- What interests you about the curriculum at [medical school]?
- Tell us what attracts you most and least about [medical school].
- What do you know about problem-based learning?
- Why do you want to come to a PBL medical school? (If relevant.)
- What do you think are the advantages and disadvantages of a PBL course? (If relevant.)
- Why do you think PBL will suit you personally? (If relevant.)

Depth and breadth of interest
- Do you read any medical publications?
- What do you think was the greatest public health advance of the twentieth century?
- Can you describe an interesting place you have been to (not necessarily medical) and explain why it was so?
- Share something that you have recently read related to the world of medicine that interested you.

Empathy
- Give an example of a situation where you have supported a friend in a difficult social circumstance. What issues did they face and how did you help them?
- How would you go about informing a patient that they have terminal cancer?
- What does the word empathy mean to you? How do you differentiate empathy from sympathy?

- What do you guess an overweight person might feel and think after being told their arthritis is due to their weight?
- A friend has asked your advice on how to tell her parents that she intends to drop out of university and go off travelling. How would you respond?

Teamwork

- Tell us about a team situation you have experienced. What did you learn about yourself and about successful team-working?
- Thinking about your membership of a team (in a work, sport, school or other setting), can you tell us about the most important contributions you made to the team?
- When you think about yourself working as a doctor, who do you think will be the most important people in the team you will be working with?
- Who are the important members of a multidisciplinary healthcare team? Why?
- Are you a leader or a follower?
- What are the advantages and disadvantages of being in a team? Do teams need leaders?

Personal insight

- Have you ever been in a situation where you realise afterwards that what you said or did was wrong? What did you do about it? What should you have done?
- How do you think doctors keep up-to-date with changes and advances during a long career?
- What are your outside interests and hobbies? Which do you think you will continue at university?
- Tell us two personal qualities you have which would make you a good doctor, and two personal shortcomings which you think you would like to overcome as you become a doctor?
- Medical training is long and being a doctor can be stressful. Some doctors who qualify never practise. What makes you think you will stick to it?
- What do you think will be the most difficult things you might encounter during your training? How will you deal with them?

Understanding of the role of medicine in society

- What is wrong with the NHS?
- What problems are there in the NHS other than the lack of funding?
- Would you argue that medicine is a science or an art, and why?
- Why do you think we hear so much about doctors and the NHS in the media today?
- In what ways do you think doctors can promote good health, other than direct treatment of illness?

- Do you think patients' treatments should be limited by the NHS budget or do they have the right to new therapies no matter what the cost?
- What do you understand by the term 'holistic' medicine? Do you think it falls within the remit of the NHS?

Work experience
- What experiences have given you insight into the world of medicine? What have you learnt from these?
- What aspect of your work experience did you find the most challenging, and why?
- Share something from your work experience or voluntary work that particularly interested you.
- Share something from your work experience that particularly shocked you.
- What aspect of your work experience would you recommend to a friend thinking about medicine, and why?
- Thinking of your work experience, can you tell me about a difficult situation you have dealt with and what you learned from it?

Tolerance of ambiguity
- Should doctors have a role in contact sports such as boxing?
- Do you think doctors should ever go on strike?
- How do you think doctors should treat injury or illness due to self-harm, smoking or excess alcohol consumption?
- Female infertility treatment is expensive, has a very low success rate and is even less successful in smokers. To whom do you think it should be available?
- Would you prescribe the oral contraceptive pill to a 14-year-old girl who is sleeping with her boyfriend?

Ethical scenarios and role plays
For each of these situations, you may be asked to explain what you would do or be expected to act it out as part of a role play.

- You are working in a café as a member of the waiting staff when a customer who is allergic to nuts brings their order back to you as they can see nuts in it. How do you respond to the customer?
- A friend tells you he feels bad because his family has always cheated to obtain extra benefits. How would you respond?
- A close friend has just split up with their partner. They are distraught and have expressed they are considering suicide. How do you deal with the situation?

Creativity, innovation and imagination
- You are going to university and you can take a suitcase with just six items in it. What would you take and why?

- Imagine a world in 200 years' time where doctors no longer exist. In what ways do you think they could be replaced?
- Is it better to give healthcare or aid to developing countries?
- Describe as many uses as you can for a mobile phone charger.
- How might you improve the process of selecting students for this medical school?
- Your house catches fire in the night. You are told you can pick only one object to take with you when escaping. What would it be and why?

Points for the interviewee to consider

In addition to your engagement with each question you are asked, it is vital that you give a generally good impression to your interviewers. You should consider these do's and don't's.

Do

- Speak clearly and at an appropriate volume.
- Answer in a friendly and positive way.
- Maintain a good degree of eye contact.
- Dress smartly. Remember it is easy to remove clothing if you feel overdressed.

Don't

- Exhibit body language tics, such as tapping your fingers on the table.
- Wear overpowering aftershave or perfume.
- Slouch in the chair.
- Swear.

You should dress smartly and sensibly for your interview, in the same way that you would for a job interview, but you should also feel comfortable.

Your aim must be to give an impression of good personal organisation and cleanliness. Make a particular point of your hair and fingernails – you never see a doctor with dirty fingernails. Always polish your shoes before an interview, as this type of detail will be noticed. Don't go in smelling strongly of aftershave, perfume or food. Make sure that you arrive early and are well prepared for the interview.

Try to achieve eye contact with each member of the panel and, as much as possible, address your answer directly to the panel member who asked the question (glancing regularly at the others), not up in the air or to a piece of furniture. Most importantly, try to relax and enjoy the interview. This will help you to project an open, cheerful personality.

Finally, watch out for irritating mannerisms. These are easily checked if you record footage of a mock interview on your phone. The interviewers will not listen to what you are saying if they are all watching to see when you are next going to scratch your left ear with your right thumb!

The interviewers

The interviewers can come from a wide variety of backgrounds, but it is likely that some of them will be academic staff from the medical school. They are often joined by medical students, practising doctors and sometimes members of the public. All interviewers are trained to apply the interview criteria accurately and fairly.

While you can expect the interviewers to be friendly, it is possible that at least one of them may come across as aggressive, angry or disinterested. Don't be put off by this; it is either an interview technique that the interviewer has been asked to adopt, or just the natural personality of the interviewer. Either way, stay positive and calm and don't deviate from how you would normally behave.

Questionnaires

An increasing number of medical schools have started to use additional forms for students to fill in with details of their work experience and personal skills. It is important to treat this even more seriously than your personal statement as it is likely to have even closer scrutiny.

A good example of this type of form is from the University of Manchester, which uses an online portal to collect information about your non-academic pursuits. This is structured in the following sections.

- Experience in a caring role.
- Hobbies and interests.
- Team working.
- Motivation for medicine.

Source: www.bmh.manchester.ac.uk/study/medicine/apply/
non-academic

Although it is likely that you will use experiences from your personal statement in these sections, it is important that they are written from scratch and not just copied straight over.

What happens next?

If your results are below the threshold score but close to it, you may be put on an official or unofficial waiting list. If you are offered a place, you will receive correspondence from the medical school telling you what you need to achieve in your A levels: this is called a conditional offer. In addition, the conditions of your offer will be added to UCAS Track, although this can take a little bit of time, so don't worry if you are made to wait a short while. Post-A level students who have achieved the necessary grades will be given unconditional offers in terms of the academic requirements, but may still be made conditional offers in relation to criminal record and health checks. If you are unlucky, all you will get is a notification from UCAS saying that you have been rejected. If this happens, it is not necessarily the end of the road in medicine, as you may be able to reapply as a post-A level applicant. What you must do in this situation is contact the universities that you applied to and ask for feedback about why you were unsuccessful. However, be warned, some universities don't give feedback, while others provide seemingly random comments that seem to bear no resemblance to your memory of the interview. Some universities will be more helpful than others and give relatively detailed feedback, which will give you points to consider.

Case study

Camrun is a second-year medical student at the University of Exeter. He arrived at his decision to study medicine following his voluntary work in Cambodia.

'I decided to study medicine after working at Khmer Sight, an ophthalmic charity based in Cambodia, for about four months. This, alongside my work experience placement at Birmingham Children's Hospital, reinforced my desire to pursue a career in medicine.

'Both of these experiences taught me how hectic and stressful medicine can be, but also how incredibly rewarding it is. Working in both Asia and the UK gave me a great insight into how the different healthcare systems work, and how grateful people can be when healthcare isn't guaranteed. I also gained some useful clinical knowledge, especially in the context of eyes.

'During my first year, I only had around five months of teaching before the pandemic hit. Since then, face-to-face teaching has been a bit hit and miss, and the majority of the work is self-directed at the moment. Even before the pandemic, I was quite surprised that medical schools take a much less active role in your learning than I was familiar with. This was especially true in clinical skills, where you are taught something and then left to your own devices to practise it and maintain a high level of proficiency, which can be quite daunting but allows you to learn quickly!

'I find the clinical aspects of the course the most interesting. In general, I have always preferred subjects that are more applied and practical than just learning the factual and theoretical side of things. There are some heavy expectations placed on you for some parts of the course, especially adapting to new styles of learning and assessment quickly, such as the Objective Structured Clinical Examinations (OSCEs), though you do so many of them over the course of the degree that you get used to them quickly. This style of learning parallels medicine and gets you used to thinking on your feet, as nothing in medicine is certain. I have really enjoyed my placements to date, and everyone is very eager to help you learn.

'At the moment, I'm not sure what I would like to specialise in. There are lots of options and I think through further placements, I will gain more insight into the possible routes for me.

'My advice for students aspiring to study medicine is not to rush into it, even if that means taking a gap year to make absolutely sure it is for you. I know for certain I wouldn't have enjoyed the course at 18 years old, but taking some time out allowed me to reflect on whether it was the right course for me, so I was more prepared when I did begin studying several years later. Lots of people feel demoralised when they are rejected during the application process, but you shouldn't let this deter you from trying. When I applied, I received a number of rejections, but managed to secure a place at Exeter. Don't worry about rejections and don't be too proud to take some time out to better yourself so you can improve your application next time around. I would also encourage applicants to practise as much as they can for UCAT, as a high score can really help with getting interviews.'

7 | Current issues

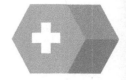

It is obviously impossible to know about all illnesses and issues in medicine. However, being aware of some of the issues in medicine today will be of enormous benefit, particularly if you are asked, as many candidates are, to extrapolate and elucidate on 'an issue' in an interview. Showing that you have an awareness of issues on more than a passing or superficial level demonstrates intelligence, interest and enthusiasm for medicine.

This will undoubtedly stand you in good stead next to a candidate who either is very hazy or is at worst completely unaware of a major issue in medicine. The following section illustrates, albeit briefly, some of the major issues that are currently causing debate, both in medical circles and in wider society. A little bit of awareness and knowledge can go a long way to securing and leaving a positive impression on an interview panel.

National Health Service (NHS)

'The NHS employs more than 1.5 million people, putting it in the top five of the world's largest workforces, together with the US Department of Defence, McDonald's, Walmart and the Chinese People's Liberation Army.'

Source: www.nhs.uk/using-the-nhs/about-the-nhs.

Since its initiation in 1948, the NHS has undergone major reforms to improve the services it provides. However, it has become a victim of its own success, and its issues are often broadcasted. The state of the NHS is a very topical issue, and one that has elicited a lot of negative comments from practitioners. It is a very common area of questioning by interview teams.

Structure of the NHS

In England, the NHS comprises a number of core organisations.

- The Department of Health and Social Care is the government department responsible for the distribution of funding for health and social care in England, as well as policy making.
- NHS England is an independent body that is not under government control. It is responsible for improving healthcare outcomes and

determining the priorities of the NHS. It is also responsible for commissioning primary care services.

- Clinical Commissioning Groups (CCGs) are statutory NHS bodies run by clinical staff, such as GPs, nurses and consultants. They play a significant role in their local area, where they commission necessary healthcare and acquire the appropriate funding. In this way, they are responsible for around 60% of the NHS budget.

NHS funding

Since the 1980s, it has been evident that as scientific advances occurred, the cost of the services provided by the NHS would continue to increase. The majority of news stories and the negativity that surrounds the NHS often come down to its chronic underfunding. In recent years, some dramatic changes have occurred in a bid to limit these pressures.

Closure of departments

In July 2012, Professor Terence Stephenson, the new chair of the Academy of Medical Royal Colleges (AoMRC), stated that many hospitals needed to close in order for there to be improvements within the NHS. He wanted ministers to downgrade NHS hospitals and rationalise intensive care units so as not to be 'wasteful' of NHS resources. He argued that by spreading themselves too thinly, doctors were not able to give the same amount of care as they would be able to do if they were concentrated in fewer locations. His arguments were designed to implement centralisation of resources.

In 2016, the picture once again was looking bleak as the NHS cut hospital units in response to the financial crisis; two hospitals had to close A&E departments for children as they could no longer run them safely. Chris Hopson, chief executive of NHS Providers, went on record saying that, 'We are reaching breaking point.'

Privatisation of the NHS

In 2012, Andrew Lansley (then secretary of State for Health) abolished the cap of 49% on private work that hospitals were allowed to do in order to secure additional funding. This opened the way for 100% privatisation of the NHS, with hospitals able to raise all of their income from private healthcare. NHS trusts were required to become self-governing by 2014. However, by September 2014, figures published showed that, instead of successful privatisation, the NHS was nearly £1 billion in debt.

The next stage was devolution and the transferral of budgets to external governing bodies. In 2016, many services were being taken over by external suppliers, for example, the Virgin Care Group, which in part had a positive effect as the debt was taken on by alternative providers; at the same time, though, such takeovers were lambasted by those that believed the new clinical commissioning groups' would focus on profits and thus destabilise local hospitals.

> **Things to consider**
>
> Most people will automatically oppose privatisation of the NHS, as they see it as a detraction from one of the NHS's core principles: free healthcare at the point of use. There are some arguments surrounding privatisation, and it is worth you familiarising yourself with them. You might want to consider the following.
>
> - Fairness – privatisation of the NHS may ultimately result in some provisions only being available to those able to afford it.
> - Feasibility – when the NHS was introduced, the consequences of an ageing population were not considered, and it is now simply too expensive to run as it stands.
> - Efficiency – when compared to insurance-based health programmes that are privately run, such as those in the US, publicly funded healthcare systems are far more efficient in that considerably less money is spent per person.
> - Continuity – in some cases, continuity of care is required, or at least preferred, and this may not always be possible in privatised sectors.
> - Costs – in private healthcare, drugs and other medical interventions have varying costs, and they typically increase year on year.
> - Choices – it is possible that privatisation may lead to enhanced options regarding where a patient is treated and what that treatment might be. However, it is unlikely that such choice would be available at an equal level, and may be of greater benefit to those who are able to afford it.

Recent changes within the NHS

'Reforms so big they can be seen from space.'
NHS Chief Executive Sir David Nicholson

The NHS in 2017

A fair summary of the NHS in recent years would be that it has become a victim of its own success. No one can deny there are problems; however, a lot of these problems are because the NHS has got better at helping people, raising expectations and, perhaps unfairly, the service is judged on that.

In 2018, the NHS celebrated its 70-year anniversary, during which time medicine had been revolutionised with regard to innovation and care. Clinical outcomes were better, cancer survival rates were higher and the number of clincial commissioning groups (20 in total) moving out of special measures and improving was positive.

Nevertheless, pressures on the NHS were greater than ever in 2017. The previous budget had not provided enough money for all of the NHS departments and the Secretary of State for Health, Jeremy Hunt's divisive order to NHS bosses to continue with current waiting times was, within the service, considered unsustainable. The NHS itself in 2017 stated that it was confronting certain paradoxes.

- *'We're getting healthier, but we're using the NHS more'*. It was estimated that life expectancy had been rising by five hours a day, but alongside that the need for NHS care was more pronounced. This was largely due to the growing and ageing population, with more than half a million more people aged over 75 since 2010 and an estimated two million more by 2020.
- *'The quality of NHS care is demonstrably improving, but we're becoming far more transparent about care gaps and mistakes'*. Survival rates were better but this had raised public expectations.
- *'Staff numbers are up, but staff are under greater pressure'*. There were 8,000 more doctors and nurses working in the NHS than there were in 2014, but these staff were not spread across all departments, rather they were clustered within certain specialisms.
- *'The public are highly satisfied with the NHS, but concerned for its future'*. Independent data from the last three decades showed that the level of satisfaction and trust from the public with the NHS was at one of its highest peaks in 2017.

The NHS Five Year Forward View described three improvement opportunities: a health gap, a quality gap, and a financial sustainability gap.

Improvements made in 2017 included:

- action on prevention and public health
- plain packaging for cigarettes
- national diabetes prevention programme
- sugar tax agreed to reduce childhood obesity
- vaccination of over 1 million infants against meningitis and an additional 2 million children against flu
- public health campaigns such as 'Be Clear on Cancer' and 'Act Fast'.

The NHS in 2019

The NHS Five Year Forward View has made a positive impact on society's healthcare standards. NHS England has now written a plan, following the 70th birthday of the NHS in 2018, to sustain it for at least another decade – this is the Long Term Plan. The Long Term Plan has a greater focus on prevention over cure, and greater access to out of hours GPs and urgent care services. In summary, the Long Term Plan aims to:

- improve provision of care based on the needs of the individual patient
- improve the quality of care at GP level to reduce hospital admissions
- improve accessibility of treatment, with faster access to services and treatments and improved proximity to patients' homes

- provide online GP consultations
- improve education of patients with diseases such as diabetes, so that they can more effectively self-manage
- invest in cancer interventions, with a greater emphasis on early diagnosis for better prognostic outcomes
- increase the number of nursing undergraduate places at university.

Perhaps one of the most exciting prospects of the Long Term Plan is an accessible and rapid screening mechanism for heart disease, which is the largest global cause of mortality. This will be achieved using risk stratification, whereby patients presenting with potential risk factors, such as diabetes, high blood pressure, atrial fibrillation or even family history of cardiovascular disease, are identified and interventions are put in place. These interventions will be largely based around changes to lifestyle, though some medical interventions, such as introduction to an anticoagulation medication, may also be utilised. The main idea behind the screening process is to reduce disease progression, as well as the associated complications of treating more advanced disease; more targeted use of resources in a specialised manner; assisting patients with informed decision-making regarding their lifestyle choices; and, overall, to reduce mortality rates through early intervention.

Current issues in the NHS

As previously discussed, the NHS is ever-changing and it is impacted by a wide range of factors. It is crucial that you keep a close eye on things relating to the NHS in the news, including regulatory and structural changes, and new findings relating to specific aspects of health. Some of the most current issues at the time of writing are discussed below.

The Covid-19 pandemic

It goes without saying that the Covid-19 coronavirus pandemic has influenced every aspect of our lives, but the NHS has undoubtedly been the most heavily impacted part of the UK. It has affected people's livelihoods, job security, incomes and social lives, all of which are required for healthy living – and this is just the tip of the iceberg.

The World Health Organisation declared the outbreak of Covid-19 as a pandemic on 11 March 2020. The first cluster of cases of pneumonia with an unknown cause was reported in Wuhan City in the Hubei Province in China on 31 December 2019; the cause was identified as a novel coronavirus, SARS-Cov-2, causing the associated disease Covid-19, on 12 January 2020.

At the time of writing (January 2021), there have been over 90 million confirmed cases around the globe and over 2 million deaths, which starkly illustrates the devastating impact of a novel infection within the human population.

The source of the outbreak is thought to be zoonotic – caused by an infectious pathogen that has transferred from a non-human animal to humans – though investigations are ongoing and are as yet undetermined. After the initial cases in Wuhan, all subsequent cases are due to human-to-human transmission which is the reason behind all of the protocols that have now become part of our daily lives – wearing face masks, remaining socially distanced and, at the peaks of infection, the country going into lockdown, where the government have encouraged everyone to stay at home as much as is physically possible.

The clinical features of Covid-19?

Perhaps one of the biggest problems with Covid-19 is its presentation: it varies considerably in terms of the symptoms that people experience, and those impacted can be completely asymptomatic or hospitalised.

The common symptoms include:

- fever
- new, continuous cough
- shortness of breath
- fatigue
- loss of appetite
- loss of taste and smell

However, this list of symptoms is not exclusive, and people have also experienced sore throats, headaches, nasal congestion, diarrhoea, nausea and vomiting.

Lockdown

The first lockdown was called on 23 March 2020, when the Prime Minister, Boris Johnson, announced the restrictions live on television. The lockdown was strict and meant that individuals in the UK could only leave their homes for food, medication or to provide care for vulnerable individuals, as well as to undertake one form of exercise per day. This involved closure of schools (leading to online teaching), and even the cancellation of exams. Initially, the lockdown was only due to last for three weeks, but it was extended far beyond this, until 10 May. Another, slightly less strict lockdown was introduced in England on 5 November 2020 for 4 weeks, and at the time of writing the UK was in another strict lockdown that began on 12 January 2021 and was due to be gradually relaxed from 8 March, with the hope that all restrictions would be eased by summer 2021.

So, why are lockdowns imposed?

- To stop the spread of infection so that the number of affected individuals falls.
- To prevent the NHS from becoming overwhelmed; in the initial lockdown it was also to provide time to prepare hospitals for further admissions by accruing specialist equipment such as ventilators for those individuals most severely affected.
- To provide time for the development of treatment plans for those becoming more severely unwell.
- To allow time for the development of a successful track and trace system.

During the first lockdown, the NHS did become more equipped and significant efforts went into the development of Nightingale hospitals, which were set up as temporary Covid-19 hospitals. Though setting up additional hospitals specialised for treatment of a particular disease during a pandemic is fairly logical, the issue that has emerged is a lack of staff. In existing hospitals, many specialist staff are redeployed to Covid wards, meaning that existing practices in a wide range of specialities are stretched enormously, negatively impacting patient care in other areas.

Lockdown

Lockdowns have proved effective in reducing cases, hospitalisations and deaths. However, there are negative consequences to lockdowns.

- The economic consequences of lockdown are dire, with many people becoming unemployed.
- There are increases in reports of domestic abuse.
- Many people report a decline in their mental health.
- School closures are likely to impact student attainment, especially for those due to sit exams in 2020 or 2021.
- Illnesses going undiagnosed due to individuals' reluctance to visit GP surgeries and hospitals during lockdown.

Impact of Covid-19 on the NHS

Covid-19 has severely disrupted NHS provisions in the UK. The government and the public health workforce have put in place restrictions and measures to control the spread of the virus and protect the most vulnerable individuals in the population, but the reality is that this has been done in the midst of continuous budget reductions for the NHS. As such, in order to support an increased demand on healthcare services, healthcare provision for non-Covid-19 patients was heavily scaled back as existing staff members have been mobilised to respond to the critical needs of patients affected by the virus.

The NHS entered the pandemic on the back foot – without enough beds and staff per capita across the country. Staffing shortages were also apparent prior to the onset of the virus. NHS trusts therefore had to make large-scale changes to their services to enhance the capacity for treating patients with Covid-19. As well as the redeployment of specialist staff, thousands of patients were discharged early to free up beds and non-urgent treatment was largely postponed. A high proportion of appointments were also postponed or moved online, which is thought to have led to many health issues requiring urgent attention being missed, or treatment interventions being made too late, having an enormous negative impact on patient health.

Throughout the first lockdown period, Accident and Emergency use and admissions dropped significantly enough to raise concerns. For example, the British Heart Foundation reported that there had been a 38% drop in emergency heart surgeries in London in the second half of March, suggesting that patients were staying away for fear of contracting the virus and putting additional pressure on the NHS. NHS England were clear that cancer treatment must continue, but it has been predicted that inevitable delays and disruption to surgery and chemotherapy would result in an increase in deaths. Of course, the impact doesn't stop here – mental health, maternity services, routine immunisations in children and the management of chronic conditions are also thought to have suffered considerably.

Shielding

In order to protect the NHS, the most clinically vulnerable people were asked to shield by staying indoors and isolating entirely. Early data from the most affected countries, including China and Italy, indicated that fatalities from Covid-19 infections were more likely in those with underlying health conditions, including heart disease, lung disease and chronic obstructive pulmonary disorders (COPD), diabetes and high blood pressure. Those identified as being most at risk were contacted by the NHS. By isolating, it was hoped that they were less likely to contract the virus and, as a result, the number of patients requiring treatment in intensive care would remain manageable.

Alarmingly, the Covid-19 deaths highlighted the disparities between the health of populations in different parts of the country. Not all elderly people, for example, were affected in the same way, and those living in more socially and economically deprived areas saw higher death rates. Similarly, there was a disproportionate impact on black, Asian and minority ethnic communities in the UK.

Future challenges

The pandemic is far from over, but already there are concerns about the reinstatement of routine care. The NHS aims for a waiting time of no more than 18 weeks, yet before the virus had reached the UK, around 730,000 individuals had been on a waiting list for a longer duration than this for routine hospital appointments, with over 4 million on the waiting list in total. With all routine appointments delayed for three months from

April 2020, the pandemic is likely to increase waiting lists even further, which will inevitably have a knock-on effect on all subsequent cases. Without significant interventions through increased funding, capacity and staffing levels, the impact could last for many years. Radical change to the delivery of routine care is to be expected in the coming years.

The Government's handling of the pandemic

In general, the Government's handling of the pandemic has drawn considerable criticism at all stages. In many cases, decisions about restrictions being put in place came much later than those in other countries with comparable infection figures, with the general perception being that needless deaths were caused by their belatedness. It was also felt by many that – as restrictions did ultimately result in bringing down case numbers, hospital admissions and the death toll – restrictions were lifted too soon and too dramatically, which ultimately led to further waves of infections.

Early on in the initial lockdown, it became apparent that there was not a sufficient amount of PPE for NHS and care workers, and millions of pounds were spent acquiring face masks that were unusable. Advice was issued to frontline staff to wash and reuse PPE where necessary, which was regarded as a wholly inappropriate action. The general feeling was that NHS staff who were risking their own health and lives were being heavily let down.

There were also several occasions where members of the Government breached lockdown rules, undermining public trust in their efforts to enforce national lockdown. Perhaps the most damaging breach was the Dominic Cummings scandal, where Boris Johnson's chief aide drove to County Durham while unwell with Covid-19 at the height of the first wave, breaking several of the rules that the Government had put in place. Johnson's support of his aide, who claimed he acted 'reasonably', caused significant controversy among the British public, with many calling for Cummings' resignation.

A positive and welcome response was the introduction of a number of economic support schemes, including the Furlough Scheme (where the Government paid 80% of wages to those staff who were temporarily surplus to workplace requirements) and Self-Employed Income Support Scheme. These measures provided financial security to many in times of profound economic uncertainty. In addition, the Government provided funding for the development of Covid-19-specific Nightingale hospitals.

Herd immunity

Early on in the pandemic, Sir Patrick Vallance, the Government's chief scientific adviser, stated that transmission would be best reduced through the development of herd immunity. Herd immunity (discussed on page 144 in the context of vaccinations) requires a large proportion of the population to become immune to an infectious agent, typically through a vaccination programme. However, as the coronavirus responsible for Covid-19 was novel, there was no vaccine, and the Government's early plans were to allow over 60% of the population to become infected with a virus with potentially devastating consequences. Understandably, this approach was heavily criticised, and the UK ultimately opted for a different approach.

Sweden was one country that adhered to the idea of natural herd immunity, without enforcing any national lockdowns, instead relying on voluntary social distancing, including working from home and avoiding public transport. In Sweden, other restrictions were also put in place, including banning large gatherings and restricted access to hospitality. The reasoning was that the restrictions would be long term and as such, this approach would be more manageable. Sweden's rates of infection have remained comparable to other European countries that have more restrictive measures in place, without the devastating impact to Sweden's economy. However, while their approach was successful early on, death rates peaked in later months, with the Swedish population rapidly losing trust in their government's handling of the situation. Similarly, despite their approach, Sweden did not achieve herd immunity, with only 7% of the population possessing antibodies by the end of April – figures comparable to Spain and France, which both had prolonged lockdowns – though the complexities in assessing this have to be acknowledged.

Things to consider

- The impact of Covid-19 in care homes – mortality rates were extremely high where care homes saw outbreaks due to the vulnerability of residents.
- Black, Asian and minority ethnic individuals were more affected by Covid-19 at its peak – this corresponded to black, Asian and minority ethnic workers making up a large proportion of key workers, but also leads to questions about institutional racism.
- The decline in the use of emergency care and how this has led to increased deaths in non-Covid-19 situations.
- The differing abilities of different regions to handle the demands of Covid-19 infections, due to differences in critical care facilities (i.e. intensive care beds were more available in London than other, particularly rural, areas).
- The loss of primary care through GPs and its negative impact on the management of chronic conditions – with many appointments being online or over the phone, communication became inaccessible for some people, with important signs and symptoms being missed.
- The provision of mental health care declined and, where it remained, it predominantly moved to online or phone appointments, which prevented many people from making use of them due to a lack of privacy when confined to the family home.

- Economic and social impacts of lockdown and social distancing measures are likely to have enduring mental health effects.
- The effectiveness of restrictions such as lockdowns and social distancing for those living in more socially and economically deprived areas, especially with lower incomes and overcrowding, which highlights significant health inequalities in the UK.
- The weaknesses of the NHS that were highlighted by the pandemic – a lack of funding, staffing shortfall and lack of specialist equipment.
- As well as disparities between regions of the UK, different countries around the world were impacted differently, with those with greater economic stability (and related benefits such as better nutrition and housing conditions) and solid borders faring better.
- Sweden's response: it did not enforce a national lockdown yet did not observe the consequences anticipated by the UK.

Useful websites

- NHS: www.nhs.uk/conditions/coronavirus-covid-19
- World Health Organisation: www.who.int/emergencies/diseases/novel-coronavirus-2019
- Statista: www.statista.com/topics/5994/the-coronavirus-disease-covid-19-outbreak
- BBC: www.bbc.co.uk/news/coronavirus

Remember that when reading about the pandemic in the media, you should consider investigating different news sources to ensure that your understanding is unbiased.

Brexit

The NHS became a political battleground once again in 2016 as the Brexit vote loomed large. The Brexit campaign will be synonymous with the image of Boris Johnson on his battle bus, with the slogan, 'We send £350 million a week to the EU. Let's fund our NHS instead.' However, the slogan, like the promise, has transpired to be misleading, and the £350 million promised during the EU referendum is unlikely to materialise.

So, what is the likely impact of Brexit on the NHS?

- New customs checks at the border and paperwork could mean potential delays and complications, at least initially.
- An end to mutual recognition of professional qualifications, although the UK has decided to continue to recognise EEA qualifications for up to two years, but there is no reciprocity. This could further impact on the NHS's current staffing problems.
- EU/EEA students are now classed as international students for fee purposes and can no longer benefit from domestic student fees

and financial support. This may deter outstanding students in medicine, nursing, midwifery and other related healthcare fields from studying and working in the UK.

Fortunately, the UK will be able to participate in the EU's scientific research and innovation programme, Horizon Europe, and the new points-based immigration system for people wanting to come and work in the UK is unlikely to exclude most healthcare workers (although care workers will be adversely affected).

Seven-day NHS

One of the most controversial issues of 2015 and 2016 was Jeremy Hunt's proposals for weekend working by doctors and consultants, which included seven-day contracts and a cut in overtime pay. However, this was not a new issue. It has been debated for the last 20 years.

The contract agreed by the Labour government had allowed consultants to opt out of non-emergency work outside of 7am–7pm from Monday to Friday. However, Jeremy Hunt argued patients were 15% more likely to die if admitted on a Sunday than midweek. He also emphasised the fact that the salaries of 40,000 consultants had been rising since 2001. Under Hunt's plans, therefore, there would be a new central contract that would mean GP practices would open, senior consultants would be on call at weekends and hospitals would have services and clinics seven days a week, rather than five days a week.

The issue, as far as the BMA was concerned, was not a lack of support for this scheme and for an improvement in the service, but rather a lack of available resources to make this plan realistic and not stretch the NHS too thin. The government wanted GP practices and hospital services available on weekends; the profession questioned the need, saying that it needed to be funded properly.

A leaked NHS memo has shown that the profession is particularly concerned about the impact of Brexit on seven-day services because of the possible demands that will be imposed on a dwindling workforce. This is among an array of other concerns the profession has about this plan.

Junior doctor contracts

The debate surrounding junior doctor contracts began in 2013. In short, the Department of Health amended contracts, which influenced pay and shift patterns. While the changes were intended to make pay fairer and provide a better service to patients, junior doctors disagreed and the British Medical Association initiated negotiations. The consequences were messy, and resulted in numerous strikes.

Initially, junior doctor contracts stipulated:

- junior doctors were to work shifts between 7am and 7pm
- a basic salary which would increase with experience
- junior doctors were expected to work some additional shifts outside of these hours
- any shifts in unsociable hours warranted additional banded pay.

Changes to contracts meant that:

- pay would be reflected by the level of training they were currently undertaking
- additional pay for on-call shifts would be linked to this level, rather than the time worked
- shifts could be worked at any time, including unsociable hours.

Junior doctors rejected these contracts for a number of reasons.

- They would be expected to work unsociable hours without financial remuneration.
- Since junior doctors would be working longer hours in unsociable shift patterns, it would be likely to cause increased stress and tiredness, making mistakes more likely and increasing the risk of jeopardy to patient care.
- The contracts would minimise the ability of doctors to change specialities once trained, since their pay would fall back down the scale to reflect their trainee status, which would mean that some areas of medicine might be underserved.
- Trainee doctors would not be able to undertake paid academic research, which could hinder individual careers as well as research progression as a whole.
- Maternity leave was not covered in initial drafts of the contract, which led to questions over equality.

Prior to these changes being made, tens of thousands of junior doctors went on strike over ongoing disputes. The BMA, which represents around 30,000 medics, said that about 76% of its members turned out to vote and of those who voted, 98% were in favour of the walkout. The BMA's Junior Doctors Committee (JDC) had planned to hold three five-day walkouts between October and December 2016, but this was called off by the BMA in September 2016, with patient safety cited as the principal concern; nonetheless, the BMA was still vocal in voicing its opposition to the introduction of the new contract. The strikes called into question the moral grounds for abandoning sick patients to protest.

The new terms and conditions for doctors (and dentists) in training in England, published in March 2018, are available to view on the NHS

Employers website at www.nhsemployers.org/-/media/Employers/Documents/Pay-and-reward/Junior-Doctors/Pay-and-Conditions-Circular-MD-12017-MARCH-2018.pdf. The new contract is in operation as of 7 August 2019: www.bma.org.uk/collective-voice/influence/key-negotiations/terms-and-conditions/junior-doctor-contract-negotiations.

Things to consider

- What do you think the ethical implications are over walkouts?
- In what situations is a strike justifiable?
- What alternative measures can you think of instead of invoking the right to strike?

Black, Asian and Minority Ethnic Communities

The Covid-19 pandemic brought to light a startling statistic – the mortality and morbidity of the virus was heavily skewed towards black, Asian and minority ethnic groups (BAME) among both staff and patients. The NHS recognised this as 'not just an equality, diversity and inclusion issue' but an 'urgent medical emergency' that required immediate action. In May 2020, the Chief Medical Officer asked Public Health England to explore the impact of Covid-19 across different population groups through analysis of various factors, such as confirmed cases, hospitalisations and deaths by ethnicity. They are focusing on several key areas.

- Protection of staff through thorough risk assessments, with an emphasis on the mental and physical health of BAME staff.
- Increased engagement with BAME staff to learn from their lived experience.
- BAME representation in decision-making processes.
- Emphasis on the rehabilitation and recovery of BAME staff through ongoing support to meet emotional needs.

While Covid-19 may have brought these issues to the fore, they have been deep rooted for a long time. Very few board members are from BAME backgrounds, and a lack of diversity at senior levels has resulted in white applicants being 1.46 times more likely to be appointed than their BAME peers. To overcome this, institutional racism and unconscious bias need to be addressed, and the NHS have set out to achieve this through the steps outlined above, but predominantly through increased BAME representation at all levels throughout the workforce and increased reflection on the experiences of BAME communities to learn from their experiences.

Social media in medicine

It is a brave new world, and it was only a matter of time before social media and medicine found a common ground. There is an increasing trend now for the use of social networking devices in order to help patients. The latest innovation is being able to get an appointment with a GP via an app on your phone; Push Doctor and Now GP are the two leading services to do this, reportedly being able to reach over 1 million patients. This reduces waiting times and gains quicker access to doctors. Only the future will show whether this will prove as effective as seeing a GP in person.

This concept has also extended into hospitals, where a Virtual Fracture Clinic is in operation at hospitals such as the Brighton and Sussex group of hospitals in order to assess more minor injuries over the phone and then refer the patient to the virtual fracture clinic for physiotherapy exercises and monitoring, thus reducing the waiting lists of those in the hospitals waiting for appointments.

Mental health

Owing to an increased awareness of mental health conditions, they are being diagnosed more frequently, and account for approximately 28% of the total burden of disease. In 2019, 5,691 suicides were registered in the UK, with men being three times more likely to take their own lives than women in the UK. As these numbers continue to rise, there has been a multitude of mental health campaigns, both by charities and Public Health England. Irrespective of how successful these campaigns are in encouraging people to seek the help that they need, the support is not always freely available through the NHS.

There is no parity between provisions for the treatment of mental and physical health conditions; just 13% of the NHS's budget is given to mental health care. Despite mental health issues being a growing concern, NHS mental health services have been reduced in a number of regions. As such, those suffering with mental health conditions, especially young people, are being failed by the NHS due to long waiting lists or a complete absence of available options.

According to the Mental Health Foundation, the most commonly diagnosed mental health problems are:

- anxiety
- depression
- bipolar disorder
- schizophrenia
- stress.

CCGs have been called into question regarding their funding allocations for mental health provisions. At present, the NHS is rolling out significant changes that should ultimately improve the landscape.

- An increase in the provision of psychological therapies, such as cognitive behavioural therapy.
- The development of digital therapies, which can be accessed rapidly.
- Improved support for high risk groups including children and young people and pregnant or new mothers.
- Reducing the travel requirements by increasing care availability closer to home.
- The introduction of specialist mental health care in A&E departments nationally.
- More thorough physical health checks for mental health patients.
- The introduction of specialist mental health services for veterans.

In recent years, there has been a huge movement around the theme of mindfulness, which is a way of managing thought processes and feelings and ultimately, mental health. Mindfulness exercises allow an individual to focus on the present moment and are a recommended treatment for those with mental health conditions. There are numerous approaches, including yoga, meditation and breathing techniques. The Mental Health Foundation, in partnership with Be Mindful, has produced an online course in mindfulness.

Public Health England is currently running a campaign called Every Mind Matters, which outlines the things that individuals can do to help manage their own mental health, as well as pointing people in the direction of information about different mental health issues, and where to get support. It also promotes the production of an 'action plan', which involves taking minor actions to improve mental health, such as:

- being more active
- undertaking social interaction
- reframing unhelpful thoughts
- being mindful, or in the present
- developing good sleep habits
- being in control of your day
- minimising worries
- carrying out self-care
- getting help and support where required.

TIP!

Public Health England runs a number of campaigns to address wider healthcare issues. It is worth keeping up to date with current campaigns, either by taking note of advertisements or looking at their website.

> **Things to consider**
>
> - The burden of mental health conditions should not be underestimated.
> - Mental health problems can be associated with a number of physical health problems.
> - Either in conjunction with their associated physical health problems or independently, mental health problems contribute enormously to absenteeism.
> - An individual's mental health is equally as important as their physical health, and NHS provisions should reflect this.

Vaccinations

A large focus of the NHS is preventative medicine. One of the ways in which the spread of disease can be minimised is through the use of vaccination. The basis of vaccination is that by introducing a weakened form of the pathogen into the body of an individual, their immune system will generate a full-blown response. In the case of infection by the live pathogen, the immune system will be in place to prevent the development of disease. As such, vaccines can present a straightforward way of minimising the spread of preventable disease. Time and money are put into vaccination programmes for a number of reasons.

- Vaccines prevent infection with diseases that can be fatal, thereby providing a successful means of saving lives.
- All vaccines are thoroughly tested for safety before being used on a large scale.
- They are regarded as being completely safe for widespread use.
- While adverse reactions, such as allergies, are possible, they are incredibly rare.
- Vaccination programmes allow for 'herd immunity'; by vaccinating the majority of a vulnerable population, the pathogen responsible for causing disease will have difficulty spreading from person to person.
- Vaccines can protect future generations, as a vaccinated mother cannot pass an infection on to her unborn child.
- Successful vaccination programmes can eradicate disease, as was the case with smallpox.
- Vaccines are more cost-effective than the treatment and management of disease caused by the infection that is being prevented.

Despite strong scientific evidence suggesting that, for the most part, vaccines are safe and effective, there has been a large movement in recent years of 'anti-vaxxers', who completely disagree with the notion of vaccination, citing numerous reasons.

- Vaccines can cause serious and, in some cases, fatal side effects.
- Vaccines can contain potentially harmful chemical compounds, such as heavy metal traces, or ingredients that some individuals see as being immoral, such as animal products.
- Vaccines cannot be mandatory, as this infringes upon human rights.
- Natural immunity is more robust than vaccines, which are unnatural.
- Vaccines target diseases which, owing to previously successful vaccination programmes, have been almost eradicated.
- In some cases, the diseases that the vaccines protect against are relatively harmless, and carry less risk than the vaccine.

One of the major contributors to the anti-vaxxer movement was the controversy associated with the combined measles, mumps and rubella (MMR) vaccine. Each infection is highly contagious and can lead to significant complications, such as deafness, encephalitis and meningitis, as well as miscarriage in pregnancy. The side effects of the MMR vaccine were mild compared to vaccinating for each disease independently, and after its introduction in 1988, the number of cases of each disease dropped considerably.

However, in 1998, Dr Andrew Wakefield published a study in *The Lancet*, a highly respected and peer-reviewed medical journal, linking the MMR vaccine to the development of autism in children. The media went to town with this information, scaring the uninformed masses into retreating from the vaccination programme. The consequences were that there was an increase in measles, mumps and rubella.

Since the publication, it was found that Dr Wakefield had fabricated the results and his work has been entirely discredited. In addition, he was banned from working as a doctor in the UK because of his falsifications. Subsequent studies conducted on a much larger scale have found no link between the MMR jab and autism. Despite this, the legacy of the work still stands, and many people still believe that there is a link.

In November 2018, Professor Dame Sally Davies, the former chief medical officer for England, encouraged parents to ignore the myths spread on social media by anti-vaccine campaigners, branding it as 'fake news'. The number of individuals vaccinated currently sits at 87%, which falls significantly short of the 95% required for herd immunity.

Things to consider

Typically, people have a specific opinion and are either fully for or against vaccination. For medical school interviews, it is worth researching these points in greater depth so that you can confidently talk through both sides of the argument. It is worth remembering that it is the right of the parent or guardian to decide whether or not children are vaccinated.

Dementia

'Dementia is set to be the 21st century's biggest killer. It is the only leading cause of death that we can't cure, prevent or slow down.'

Alzheimer's Society

Dementia is a collective term for a group of brain disorders that result in a progressive loss of brain function. Among the diseases described by dementia, Alzheimer's disease is the most common, with between 50–75% of diagnosed individuals affected by it. Over the last few years, the term 'dementia' has been used far more frequently by the media, and this can be attributed to the vast increase in the number of diagnosed cases and resulting deaths.

Different forms of dementia

There are numerous different forms of dementia, including:

- Alzheimer's disease
- vascular dementia
- dementia with Lewy bodies
- frontotemporal dementia.

It can also arise from more rare conditions, such as:

- Huntington's disease
- corticobasal degeneration
- progressive supranuclear palsy
- normal pressure hydrocephalus.

You are not expected to have a great deal of understanding about the biological basis of dementia in each of these diseases, but it is worth considering that the progression of each disease differs significantly, making it harder to diagnose and treat each individual.

Why are the numbers increasing so drastically?

In 2017, dementia and Alzheimer's disease were once again the leading cause of death in the UK according to the Office for National Statistics, accounting for 12.7% of recorded deaths. There are thought to be around 850,000 living with a form of dementia in the UK, with the number of cases expected to exceed one million by 2025. Reasons for this include the following.

- An ageing population – individuals now have a longer life expectancy, and dementia is more common in elderly people.

- Better healthcare provisions for other leading causes of death – cardiovascular disease, among other leading causes of death, can now be treated and managed more effectively, which is reducing the death toll for these diseases.
- Greater awareness – dementia is now being cited as a cause of death more frequently owing to an improved understanding of the disease by healthcare professionals.

At present, there is no cure for the different forms of dementia. A huge focus of healthcare professionals at the moment is prevention of the disease, or at least delaying the onset in those at high risk.

Some of the risk factors for dementia include:

- age – dementia is more likely to develop in older age
- genetic predisposition – there are a number of gene variants that are thought to be linked with the onset of dementia.

New research has also linked the following to the onset of dementia:

- lower levels of education
- hearing loss
- untreated depression
- social isolation
- sedentary lifestyles.

Lifestyle medicine, a term used with a much higher frequency of late, is being branded as a means of reducing the risk of developing a number of diseases, including those encompassed by dementia. The logic is that a healthy lifestyle, as reflected by a balanced diet (which is high in fibre, and low in saturated fat, salt and sugar), maintaining a healthy weight, regular exercise, stopping smoking and minimising alcohol intake, is likely to prevent disease from occurring. By the time that diagnosis has occurred, the damage to the brain is too significant to reverse, which is why the focus is on early intervention.

In the context of the pandemic, the high incidence of dementia in the UK population takes on even more significance: the Office for National Statistics reported in May 2020 that dementia is the main underlying condition for Covid-19 deaths, with 25.3% of the deaths in March and April occurring in patients with dementia and Alzheimer's in England and Wales. Perhaps more alarmingly, deaths attributed to dementia alone (without Covid-19) during April 2020 increased dramatically, with an 80% increase in England and 50% in Wales, highlighting the impact that the pandemic has had on other areas of healthcare.

> **In the news**
>
> In November 2018, headlines appeared in the media reporting that a simple neck scan could identify those at risk of dementia prior to the onset of symptoms. It came as a result of a study conducted by University College London, which measured the intensity of the pulse carrying blood towards the brain in over 3,000 people.
>
> - An ultrasound scan of the neck was carried out on each individual.
> - Stronger pulses were associated with damage to the small blood vessels supplying the brain.
> - The consequence of this damage is structural changes to the blood vessel network in the brain, as well as 'mini strokes', or minor bleeds on the brain.
> - All of the participants were then monitored over a 15-year period by assessing their memory and ability to solve problems.
> - The results indicated that those with stronger pulses at the beginning of the study were 50% more likely to show accelerated cognitive decline, which is an early indicator of dementia.
>
> While cognitive decline is a strong indicator of dementia, not everyone who experiences it is ultimately diagnosed with a dementia-related disease. However, since the development of dementia is exacerbated considerably by lifestyle factors, early interventions such as improving diet, introducing exercise and stopping smoking can minimise the chances of it occurring in individuals with more intense neck pulses.

Air pollution

Air pollution is classified as the introduction of harmful or excessive quantities of substances into the Earth's atmosphere, such as gases, particulate matter and biological molecules. Breathing is absolutely vital to staying alive, but walking along a busy city street makes that crucial act incredibly risky. With 91% of the world's population living in an area where air pollution levels exceed World Health Organization limits, it's no wonder that the health implications are becoming an increasing concern. The statistics show that most countries are at risk of the consequences of air pollution, but the most significant burden is in low- and middle-income countries.

> **What are the pollutants?**
> - Particulate matter
> - Ozone
> - Nitrogen dioxide
> - Sulphur dioxide

On average, 4.2 million deaths worldwide are attributed to ambient air pollution each year. These are predominantly a result of:

● lung cancer
● respiratory infections
● stroke
● heart disease
● chronic obstructive pulmonary disease (COPD).

Both child and adult health can be impaired by air pollution, whether it is either short- or long-term. Most commonly, it is associated with compromised lung function, more frequent respiratory infections and aggravation of conditions such as asthma. In addition, exposure to air pollution in expectant mothers is thought to lead to adverse outcomes at birth.

In the UK, the Department for Environment, Food and Rural Affairs provides guidelines to minimise the impact of air pollution at peak times, especially in high risk groups. Some examples include:

● reducing levels of outdoor exercise when pollution levels are high
● limited exertion on high pollution days in the elderly and those with heart and lung conditions
● continuing the use of medication as advised by healthcare practitioners in asthmatics, and increasing the use of inhaled reliever medication where required.

The department's advice is summarised in Table 7 on page 150.

The World Health Organization published a roadmap in 2016, outlining key areas that it plans to address in the near future.

● Improving public knowledge of the impacts of air pollution on health.
● Improving the reporting on health trends associated with air pollution.
● Improved utilisation of the healthcare sector to meet the above targets locally, nationally, regionally and globally.

In addition, a number of Sustainable Development Goals have been put in place. Essentially, these are a list of targets put in place to improve global health in relation to air pollution.

● A significant decrease in the reduction of air pollution-related deaths and illnesses.
● Access to clean energy in homes to reduce the output of air pollution.
● Access to sustainable, safe and affordable transport methods.
● Reducing the environmental impact of cities.

It is worth researching what is being done in your city to meet these goals. In the UK, local councils are integrating ways to reduce air

Table 7 DEFRA guidelines

Air Pollution banding	Value	Accompanying health messages for at-risk groups and the general populace	
		At-risk individuals	General population
Low	1-3	**Enjoy** your usual outdoor activities.	**Enjoy** your usual outdoor activities.
Moderate	4-6	Adults and children with lung problems, and adults with heart problems, **who experience symptoms**, should **consider reducing** strenuous physical activity, particularly outdoors.	**Enjoy** your usual outdoor activities.
High	7-9	Adults and children with lung problems, and adults with heart problems, should **reduce** strenuous physical exertion, particularly if they experience symptoms. People with asthma may find they need to use their reliever inhaler more often. Older people should **reduce** physical exertion.	Anyone experiencing discomfort such as sore eyes, cough or sore throat should **consider reducing** activity, particularly outdoors.
Very high	10	Adults and children with lung problems, adults with heart problems, and older people, should **avoid** strenuous physical exertion. People with asthma may find they need to use their reliever inhaler more often.	**Reduce** physical exertion, particularly outdoors, especially if you experience symptoms such as cough or sore throat.

Source: https://uk-air.defra.gov.uk/air-pollution/daqi?view=effects.
Available under the Open Government Licence v3.0

pollution. For example, Birmingham City Council recently introduced the concept of a 'Clear Air Zone', or CAZ, from June 2021. The idea is that polluting vehicles must pay to use major roads to enter the city centre, with a view to deterring people from using vehicles that do not meet specific pollution standards and to encourage them to make use of public transport instead. The reliance on individual local authorities to take action has been viewed as insufficient however, and companies such as ClientEarth have repeatedly taken the UK government to court regarding these inadequacies.

Irrespective of the effectiveness of these interventions, there is no doubt that the developed world is trying to improve this situation owing to an improved understanding of its impact on health. As promising as this is, the developing world is getting worse, and air pollution is now regarded as a public health emergency.

In the news

Claims that childhood obesity is linked to air pollution made the headlines in November 2018. The results of a study that looked at over 2,000 children in southern California found that exposure to high levels of nitrogen dioxide in the first year of life was associated with more significant weight gain during childhood. The study's results supported those of additional recent research into the impact of air pollutants and obesity. The study:

- looked at the impact of air pollution from busy main roads
- found that children who were exposed to high amounts of nitrogen dioxide were, on average, around 1kg heavier by age ten than those with minimal exposure to air pollution
- was careful to monitor other factors that could impact weight gain, including diet, gender and parental education.

While a possible link between obesity in childhood and air pollution has been demonstrated, further research must be conducted into the biological mechanisms that underpin how inhaled substances can influence the process of fat storage.

Case study

In February 2013, nine-year-old Ella Kissi-Debrah tragically passed away from a fatal asthma attack. Ella lived in close proximity to one of London's busiest roads, and had been hospitalised 27 times in the three years preceding her death. In 2019, a new inquest into Ella's death was initiated to investigate whether unlawful levels of air pollution were a contributing factor. In a landmark case, the coroner concluded that Ella died from acute respiratory failure, asthma and "air pollution exposure". This is the first time that air pollution has been declared as a contributory cause of illness and death.

Personalised medicine

The current approach to medicine is, for the most part, 'one size fits all': once a patient is diagnosed with a condition, they might be given a drug or a treatment programme that is generic to that particular disease.

However, with most conditions, there are individual cases where the method of treatment is ineffective and, for a long time, this was put down to individual differences that could not be helped.

One such example is the treatment of heart disease (or more specifically, coronary artery disease) by a drug known as clopidogrel, which prevents the formation of blood clots. In 2010, clopidogrel was the second most widely prescribed drug in the USA, despite reports of marked variability between patient responses. In short, doctors were aware that the drug might not be effective, but as it was still the most effective treatment available, they prescribed it anyway.

Fast forward several years and countless studies later, and scientists have pinpointed the reason for its outstanding effectiveness in some patients and the complete lack of impact in others. The drug works by targeting a specific enzyme in the liver, but due to genetic differences between individuals, the structure of these enzymes can differ significantly. If a patient does not have the specific enzyme that clopidogrel acts upon, it will not work, and they are still at an extremely high risk of having a heart attack.

Understanding the mechanism of action of the drug and the varied responses was incredibly important, but it led to a bigger question: what can be done about this clinically? A genetic test emerged and was utilised by some private healthcare companies in the USA that, in a couple of hours, allowed doctors to see whether or not the drug would be effective. For numerous reasons, such as the tests available being in their early stages and a lack of large-scale studies and clinical trials, these specific tests have not been rolled out nationally or globally just yet. However, it nicely outlines the basis of precision medicine.

Precision medicine is a movement that is working towards the better management of patient health by ascertaining individual differences and using therapies that are targeted to them directly. Ultimately, this should result in improved health outcomes and an overall reduced cost of healthcare owing to the improved specificity of the treatments provided.

The concept of personalised medicine has been around for a long time, but it is advances in technology that are allowing for the identification of useful interventions, and even whether an individual is at risk of developing a particular disease.

The four Ps of personalised medicine

The NHS has outlined the advantages of personalised medicine as 'the four Ps', which are summarised below.

1. **Prediction and prevention of disease.** New technologies will allow for the identification of diagnostic markers that indicate an individual

is likely to develop a particular disease, even before they show symptoms. This could allow for advice to be given on adopting better lifestyle choices, and provide an opportunity for early treatment.

2. **Precise diagnosis.** Two patients diagnosed with the same disease as they have the same symptoms may not necessarily mean that the cause of their disease is the same. As such, personalised medicine will allow for each individual's molecular and cellular processes to be carefully analysed, so that the specific nature of their disease can be understood.

3. **Personalised interventions.** As the origin of the disease can be identified, treatment methods can also be provided in a very specific manner. This could be through the prescription of a specific drug, or even a point-of-care genetic test to establish what the best treatment option might be. In doing so, the NHS will be able to move away from the 'trial and error' approach to treating disease, which is costly and can result in adverse drug responses.

4. **Participation of patients.** By improving understanding, doctors can talk to patients about what they can do to help themselves. In many diseases, improving lifestyle factors can prevent the onset of a disease that they are predisposed to, or help with the management of a disease with which they have already been diagnosed.

In light of the enormous funding pressures on the NHS, the introduction of personalised medicine could assist with the alleviation of resource allocation issues. While the integration of technologies may be costly initially, in the long term, the costs of diagnosis and treatment will be much reduced, as less money will be wasted on inefficient treatments and unnecessary diagnostic tests.

The science of genomics

The movement of genomics – a term relating to the science of genetics, but using advanced technology – has really paved the way for personalised medicine and underpins every aspect of it.

The Human Genome Project, completed in 2003, was an enormous undertaking that involved the collective efforts of scientists globally over a 15-year period and, at the time, cost an extortionate $3 billion. Nowadays, a whole human genome can be sequenced in a matter of hours for less than £1000, and these prices continue to fall. It is these technological advances that have made the possibility of sequencing each individual genome a reality.

The sequencing of whole genomes is referred to as Whole Genome Sequencing (WGS), and there are many institutions worldwide that have conducted large scale projects. In the UK alone there are many significant projects, but the one that has had the largest impact to date is the 100,000 Genomes Project.

The 100,000 Genomes Project

The 100,000 Genomes Project was initiated by former Prime Minister David Cameron, who allocated funding to the project in 2012 for the sequencing of 100,000 genomes of NHS patients and their relatives who were affected by rare and poorly understood genetic diseases and cancers. The initial aims of the project were to identify the causes of rare diseases and allow new medical research to take place to identify treatments and cures for what are typically fatal and devastating conditions. The 100,000th sequence was achieved in December 2018. Now, the project aims to support the NHS with improved treatment of conditions as it moves towards an era of personalised medicine.

Despite the enormous promise that projects such as the 100,000 Genomes Project and the notion of personalised medicine present, there are some reservations.

- Genomics is an enormous data science – that is to say, vast quantities of personal data, in the form of genomes, are being stored and obtained for free. There are concerns about the safety of that data, or even that there may be commercial gain for companies from information that has been provided by patients for free.
- Ethical concerns – some issues have been raised about the knowledge of the state of a patient's health. Some concerns have been raised over whether or not patients should be given information about additional potential health problems revealed by their genome (for example, if a doctor is looking to establish which treatment is best for a heart condition, and discovers that the patient is also likely to develop a particular form of cancer).

In the news

In July 2018, headlines stated that a new, routine DNA test will put the NHS at the forefront of medicine. The tests referred to in the headline are routine genomic tests for individuals diagnosed with cancer that will allow for the reading, analysis and interpretation of tumour DNA by specialist genomics centres around the UK. In doing so, the specific molecular cause of the cancer can be identified, and patients can be 'matched' with the most effective treatment, minimising adverse responses to drugs in the process. These new tests were rolled out across the UK on 1 October 2018, and look to be the first tangible step in the NHS's move towards personalised medicine.

Ageing population

Globally, life expectancy continues to rise (except in many sub-Saharan African countries, which have been ravaged by HIV/AIDS) because of improvements in sanitation and medical care. According to the WHO, the number of people aged 65 or over will almost triple by 2050, from about 524 million people in 2010 to over 1.5 billion people, which is approximately 16% of the world's population. Birth rates in most countries are falling, and the combination of the two brings considerable problems. The relative number of people who succumb to chronic illness (such as cancer, diabetes or diseases of the circulatory system) is increasing, and this puts greater strain on countries' healthcare systems.

It is a well-reported fact that the population of the UK is ageing. The Office for National Statistics (ONS) reports that 18.3% of the UK population were aged over 65 in 2018, and by 2038, this is expected to increase to 24.2%. These statistics can be attributed to the continuing developments in technology, improvements in healthcare and a better quality of lifestyle, all of which are contributing to people living longer lives.

Perhaps the most important aspects to consider are the challenges that an ageing population presents. Predominantly, these challenges come in the form of increased healthcare demands, and an associated increase in healthcare costs. This is attributable to an increase in the diagnosis of diseases that are more common in elderly people, such as dementia.

As technology and healthcare continue to improve, it is unlikely that life expectancy will fall. As such, there is a new focus by the NHS in partnership with Age UK to change the view of old age: rather than reacting to the frailty of the elderly, we must now start to take a proactive approach to reducing it.

Things to consider

It is worth considering some of the differences in life expectancy in different populations when preparing for interviews, as these differences may point you in the direction of mechanisms put in place by different healthcare systems.

- Why does Japan have the highest life expectancy?
- Why does France have a higher life expectancy than the UK?
- Why are most of the countries with the lowest Health Adjusted Life Expectancy (HALE) figures located in the middle and southern parts of Africa?

You can probably guess the answers to these, but, if not, further data is available at www.who.int/gho/en.

Lifestyle factors

Obesity

Obesity is an increasing problem throughout the UK, especially in the younger generation. With the UK at the top of the European obesity league, it is a big issue and very much an interview question. The last recorded Health Survey for England of 2017 (published in 2018) revealed that 29% of adults are clinically obese and 67% of men and 62% of women are overweight or obese. Obesity is defined as having a body mass index (BMI) of above 30. The annual cost is roughly £6–8 billion to the NHS (estimated to be £9.7 billion by 2050), and £49.9 billion to the wider economy.

The main causes of obesity are a combination of a lack of exercise and the consumption of excessive calories. Obesity has detrimental effects on many components of the human body, especially in later life. The extra body weight means the heart has to work harder and therefore there is an increase in blood pressure: this can lead to coronary heart disease. Atherosclerosis often occurs, which is a build-up of cholesterol and fatty substances in the lining of the arteries. This reduces the flow of blood and therefore oxygen to the heart muscle or other tissues such as the brain. Without oxygen even for a short time, cells in these tissues die. Obesity has also been shown, among other conditions, to cause respiratory problems, type 2 diabetes, and osteoarthritis due to the extra strain on the joints. The government produced a White Paper called *Healthy Lives, Healthy People: Our strategy for public health in England*. This paper, along with a document produced by the Department of Health, sets out how the problem of obesity will be dealt with over the coming years. Visit https://assets.publishing.service.gov.uk/government/uploads/system/uploads/attachment_data/file/216096/dh_127424.pdf for more details.

Childhood obesity

According to the government's Health Survey for England 2017, in 2017, 30% of children aged 2 to 15 years were overweight or obese, including 17% who were obese. It is a fact that children with obese parents are 12 times more likely to be obese than children with healthier parents, and almost twice as many children living in the most deprived areas were obese as those living in the least deprived areas. It is reported that a quarter of children aged 2 to 15 years spend at least six hours every weekend day being inactive. This is the highest rate in Western Europe and contributes to the estimated overall annual cost of obesity of £6–8 billion to the NHS in the UK. In order to address the dangers that obesity can have for children's health, the Chartered Society of Physiotherapy has published extensive guidelines designed to try and engage parents and young children with the idea of regular exercise in a healthy lifestyle. In light of these statistics, it is clear that this issue is immensely important in terms of both preventing our children from becoming obese as well as protecting future generations.

Why is obesity a problem?

Obesity is linked to a number of health problems, including:

- coronary heart disease (CHD)
- type 2 diabetes
- increased risk of a number of cancers
- stroke
- high blood pressure
- high cholesterol levels
- asthma
- gallstones
- sleep apnoea
- liver disease
- kidney disease
- osteoarthritis.

What is being done about it?

The government is rolling out a number of initiatives to reduce obesity, especially in children.

- The introduction of a soft drinks industry levy.
- Investment into school programmes to encourage physical activity and healthy eating.
- Reducing the sugar content of products by 20%.
- Supporting businesses to make their products healthier.
- Updating the nutrient profile model.
- Making healthy food options more readily available.
- The production of programmes to ensure that children enjoy one hour of physical activity a day.
- Improving the nutritional value of food in schools.
- Producing a healthy rating for school foods.
- Labelling food more clearly.

In addition, the NHS provides relatively easy to follow guidelines about how you can improve your lifestyle to lose weight, such as the promotion of its 'Couch to 5k' running programme. The basic advice is to eat a healthier diet and carry out 2.5 to 5 hours of exercise per week.

Things to consider

- Some causes of obesity may be medical, such as hypothyroidism, so it is important to discuss obesity with a degree of empathy.
- Doctors and other healthcare professionals play an important role in developing the knowledge of people relating to the causes of obesity; avoid stating that the NHS should focus on treating disease in an interview, as this is simply not the case.

Smoking

For a long time, smoking has been known to have a negative impact on overall health. In the UK, around 7.2 million adults smoke cigarettes, and it is the leading cause of preventable illness. Summarised below are some key statistics from 2018 (the latest available at the time of writing).

- 14.7% of adults smoke: 16.5% of men and 13% of women.
- Smoking is more common in younger people, and is highest in the 25–34 age range.
- Two-thirds of young people start smoking before the age of 18.
- Around 77,800 people died in the UK from smoking-induced diseases in 2018.
- Over one-third of respiratory-related deaths are related to smoking.
- Over one-quarter of cancer deaths are related to smoking.
- Approximately one-quarter of cardiovascular disease deaths are related to smoking.

That said, fewer than one in five persons in the UK now smoke and the smoking rate has halved since 1974 when roughly half of all men and 40% of all women smoked. This reduction is largely due to a number of measures taken to combat smoking in the past couple of decades, the most important being the ban on smoking inside public buildings, as a lot of people were suffering from second-hand smoke. In more recent years, the marketing on cigarette packaging has changed to include no branding other than a health warning. There has also been a rise in 'vaping' as an alternative to smoking.

More needs to be done though as, while the adult smoking rate is declining, other reports claim that two-thirds of smokers have smoked before they are 18, which represents a significant future health warning.

There have been some significant efforts by the NHS and Public Health England to deter individuals from smoking. You might want to look into:

- the NHS's Stop Smoking Services
- Public Health England's Stoptober campaign.

Things to consider

- The potential health implications of vaping.
- Smoking is linked to conditions such as lung cancer, dementia and coronary artery disease, but some controversial research suggests that it could reduce the risk of Parkinson's disease and obesity. Consider the implications of this information being publicly available.

Opinions should be balanced and acknowledge the preferences of everyone; don't think purely from a medical practitioner's point of view.

Artificial intelligence

Artificial intelligence is a field that incites both admiration and fear in the general population. While the risk of robots taking over is a notion that many deem as a not too distant reality, it is impossible to ignore the great advances that developments in artificial intelligence have allowed for. Artificial intelligence refers to the use of algorithms and computer software to carry out processes that typically require human cognition, such as the ability to make inferences, deductions and decisions, as well as identifying patterns and deviations. The latter is the basis of diagnosis in many cases, which demonstrates the space for artificial intelligence in medicine.

If humans trained as doctors are able to carry out these processes, why would we want to implement machines that can do it for us? There are a number of reasons, including the following.

- **Improvements in diagnosis.** Computers are able to identify more subtle variations than humans. If disease can be spotted by identifying minor changes on an x-ray before they become apparent to the human eye, for example, it can lead to an earlier diagnosis. Subsequently, interventions will be more rapid and improved.
- **Virtual investigations.** Patients can wear devices that monitor certain outputs, and these can be monitored by 'virtual nurses', or robots, which interpret the information and contact the patient in their own home. A useful example is reminding elderly patients to take their medications at specific times, which minimises lapses in health and ultimately, hospital admissions.
- **Robotic surgery.** In recent years, there has been a considerable increase in the number of routine operations that are conducted by robotic arms. On the whole, the operations are conducted effectively and are typically associated with more rapid recovery times and fewer complications.

While artificial intelligence clearly has a place in medicine, you might want to consider possible issues. At present, the general public does not seem receptive to the idea that robots should replace healthcare professionals in any context, but would reduced waiting times for seeing a GP or having an operation change their minds? Similarly, it could save the NHS a lot of money, which could then be reallocated to areas that need it more. However, this might be accompanied by a loss of jobs in the future, which is another concern.

Current use of artificial intelligence in medicine

Some of the uses of artificial intelligence that you might want to consider further include:

- the use of nanorobots for drug delivery
- the development of electronic health records
- the analysis of test results, such as medical image scans
- digital consultations
- virtual nursing
- precision medicine
- health monitoring.

Antibiotic resistance

As bacteria are finding more ways of adapting and surviving antibiotics, the effectiveness of antibiotics is decreasing at a rapid rate. Therefore, a campaign has been launched by Public Health England, called Keep Antibiotics Working, to urge patients to only use antibiotics when absolutely required; if they are used at less critical moments, the antibiotics may not be able to counteract a more virulent illness in the future. However, it is not just the responsibility of the patient to take antibiotics as prescribed (and not save them for another illness); it is also the responsibility of doctors to appropriately prescribe them, and this is currently being addressed with doctors.

Factors that have contributed to the antibiotics resistance crisis include:

- overuse of antibiotics for cases where they are not required
- antibiotics being prescribed incorrectly
- widespread use of antibiotics in agriculture
- barriers in the pharmaceutical industry.

As well as measures being put in place to prevent the worsening of the situation, a vast amount of research is being conducted into alternative drug therapies, such as the use of monoclonal antibodies, rather than the use of antibiotics. Many of the new aims of pharmaceutical development are aligned with the concept of personalised medicine.

At this time, antibiotic resistance is one of the greatest threats to the safety of patients in Europe and needs careful stewardship to ensure the effectiveness of the drugs in the next decade.

Things to consider

In recent years, there have been several outbreaks of 'incurable' infections due to the worsening of the antibiotic resistance situation. Notable cases include:

- Methicillin-resistant Staphylococcus Aureus (MRSA), which ravaged hospitals over a decade ago, but is now effectively managed
- 'Super' Gonorrhoea, which is a notable outbreak of an 'incurable' form of the sexually transmitted infection that became resistant to the commonly used antibiotic.

Top 10 causes of death in the world

Around the world, the most common causes of death vary considerably depending on the country in question. A number of factors influence the situation, such as the economic stability, geographical location and healthcare provisions. The following conditions are attributed to being the most significant causes of death globally according to the WHO in 2018, and accounted for 54% of the 56.9 million deaths that occurred in 2016.

- Ischaemic heart disease, caused by the narrowing of the coronary arteries that supply the heart muscle with blood, which was responsible for around 9.5 million deaths.
- Stroke, which arises due to a blocking of the arteries that supply the brain with blood, which was responsible for just under 6 million deaths.
- Chronic obstructive pulmonary disease (COPD), such as emphysema, asthma and bronchitis, claimed 3 million lives.
- Lower respiratory infections, such as pneumonia, were the most deadly communicable disease, causing 3 million deaths.
- Alzheimer's disease and other dementias were responsible for over 2 million deaths.
- Trachea, bronchus and lung cancers accounted for 1.7 million deaths.
- Diabetes mellitus, a chronic disease characterised by the inability to regulate blood glucose concentration, was responsible for 1.6 million deaths, which was a considerable increase since 2000.
- Road injury, which accounted for 1.4 million deaths, and almost three-quarters of the cases were male.
- Diarrhoeal diseases contributed to 1.4 million deaths, which was a considerable decrease of 1 million since the year 2000.
- Tuberculosis, an infection that predominantly affects the lungs, caused 1.3 million deaths.

Notable changes to the list of the top 10 causes of death is the removal of HIV and AIDS, as well as their related complications. This can be attributed to the improved knowledge surrounding the transmission of HIV, and individuals taking the necessary precautions, such as practising safe sex, to minimise the risk of transmission.

TIP!

It is worth looking at the ways that these diseases can be controlled, treated and prevented, highlighting any key actions that have been put in place, or any specific reasons that they cause death so frequently.

Legal cases

While medicine is a career that is incredibly rewarding, there is no doubt that it can be very stressful, and many of these situations can be attributed to the significant responsibility that a doctor carries in the care of their patients, the enormous pressures placed upon them when considering the current state of the NHS, and the questions and cases to which there are no clear answers. There have been a number of high-profile cases in recent years, and some of these are discussed below.

The Bawa-Garba case

The Bawa-Garba case is a legal case that has recently appeared in the media more frequently, despite starting in 2011. In a ruling in 2015, Dr Bawa-Garba was convicted of manslaughter on the grounds of gross negligence following the death of a patient for whom he was responsible.

- A six-year-old patient, Jack Adcock, was admitted to Leicester Royal Infirmary on 18 February 2011.
- He had Down's syndrome and a known heart condition, and reported with diarrhoea, vomiting and breathing difficulties.
- He was treated by Dr Hadiza Bawa-Garba, a specialist registrar in her sixth year of training, who had an impeccable record.
- She ordered blood tests and a chest x-ray which, when the results became available several hours later, indicated a chest infection.
- Upon reviewing the results of the x-ray, once she was informed that they were available after a delay of several hours, Dr Bawa-Garba prescribed antibiotics for the treatment of pneumonia that were later given by nurses.
- The results of the blood test, which identified the presence of C-reactive protein, an indicator of infection, were not available until much later due to a technological failing.
- When debriefing with her superior, she raised her findings but did not express major concern or ask the consultant to intervene since Jack appeared to be much improved.
- When writing up her notes, Dr Bawa-Garba failed to include that Jack's medication for his heart condition should be stopped.
- Jack was subsequently given his medication by his mother as she was unaware of this instruction.
- An hour later, a crash call went out and among other doctors, Dr Bawa-Garba responded as Jack suffered cardiac arrest.
- As she had confused Jack with another patient, she mistakenly called off resuscitation.
- The mistake was recognised shortly afterwards and resuscitation continued within a few minutes.
- Shortly afterwards, Jack passed away, though it was clear that the resuscitation error was not responsible.

Other areas worthy of consideration include the fact that Dr Bawa-Garba had recently returned from maternity leave, and this was her first shift in an acute ward since returning. Prior to that fateful day, Dr Bawa-Garba's record was outstanding. However, Dr Bawa-Garba's mistakes were not the only ones worth considering, as she was failed by the hospital itself.

Below are some of the arguments in Dr Bawa-Garba's defence.

- The understaffing of the hospital meaning that Dr Bawa-Garba was extremely overworked and conducting the work of two doctors.
- There were times during the day when, despite being a trainee herself, Dr Bawa-Garba was the most senior member of staff on the ward, so she had no one to report to.
- There was no system in the hospital for the communication of results to Dr Bawa-Garba, which delayed the treatment.
- The failing of the computer systems, which prevented Dr Bawa-Garba from getting the results of the blood test in good time.
- Dr Bawa-Garba did not administer Jack's medication for his heart condition.

Things to consider

- What are your thoughts on this? Consider the arguments from all angles.
- If the hospital was better staffed, would Jack have died?
- If the hospital computer systems had not failed, would interventions have been faster?
- Should Dr Bawa-Garba have to take full responsibility for this case?
- Were Dr Bawa-Garba's mistakes inexcusable?

In many other jobs, a series of mistakes such as these might go unnoticed, but as a doctor, the impacts will almost always be significant.

After being convicted of manslaughter, Dr Bawa-Garba had an appeal denied in 2016. There was an outcry from many doctors who felt that she was not defended appropriately, and more of an onus should have been placed on the poor working conditions in the NHS and especially, the lack of support available for junior and trainee doctors.

The failed appeal meant that Dr Bawa-Garba was struck off from the GMC register for 12 months, and this initiated a controversial series of legal events. The GMC applied to have her permanently struck off the register, but the Medical Practitioners Tribunal Services (MPTS) claimed that the punishment would be disproportionate. Unsatisfied with this response, the GMC took the MPTS to court and won, resulting in the prevention of Dr Bawa-Garba from practising medicine again. Again, this led to an enormous protest by doctors and ultimately, a crowdfunding effort that provided her with the funds to appeal her case. After a trying few years, Dr Bawa-Garba won her case, and the 12-month suspension was reinstated.

While complex, the case calls into question some of the darker aspects of working as a doctor in the NHS. As a doctor, you are responsible for your actions, even when training. For many, it is an unsettling and unpleasant side of a career in healthcare, but it is worth your reflection.

Simon Bramhall: The liver branding surgeon

Simon Bramhall was a leading surgeon in the field of liver transplantation. He was a highly regarded surgeon owing to his fastidious approach to surgery, and as a result, he had been able to save countless lives.

Following one of these life-saving operations – a perfectly executed liver transplant – a follow-up operation was required for unrelated reasons. A different surgeon conducted the operation, and on doing so, found the 'branding' of Dr Bramhall's initials on the liver of the patient. The branding process, which used an argon beam machine typically used to control bleeding during surgery, did not damage the liver in any way.

The case was taken to trial, and was the first of its kind. Dr Bramhall admitted to two counts of assault by beating and consequently resigned from his high-profile job. During the trial, it was considered that Dr Bramhall was tired and stressed, and during a period of significant cognitive overload, his judgement might be impaired. However, the act was viewed as 'arrogant', and while intended to relieve tension in an overwrought operating theatre, there were considerable ethical implications.

The end result was that Dr Bramhall was fined £10,000 and made to carry out 120 hours of unpaid community service. The case divided the public, and especially his patients; some felt abused by his misuse of power, while others stated that they would be proud to have been branded by him after he saved their lives. Irrespective of personal viewpoints, it was an important case for the NHS as it reinstated patient confidence.

Case study

Dr Simon Bramhall qualified as a doctor in 1988, and held numerous prestigious positions before becoming a high profile liver transplant specialist. The complex case discussed above impeded his career, but his reflections here are worthy of your consideration.

'Once I had qualified in 1988, I worked as a house officer at a hospital in Birmingham. I also worked as an anatomy demonstrator and during that time, I trained as a surgeon. I then worked in the accident and emergency department before undertaking a surgical house officer role. I gradually worked my way up the ladder of responsibility, working as a fellowship registrar, obtaining Fellowship of the Royal Colleges of Surgeons (FRCS). As I wasn't sure what I wanted to do at the time, I undertook a research job in the molecular study of pancreatic cancer.

'I later became a full-time lecturer in surgery and during that time, I also completed my Certificate of Completion Specialist Training (CCST). By this stage, I knew I wanted to be a liver transplant surgeon, but there were no jobs available. My post as a lecturer continued until a consultant post became available, which I was successful in obtaining. I became a high profile local, national and international liver transplant surgeon until I made a significant error during a period of enormous cognitive overload. My mistakes played out in the national and international press for a period of five years.

'During this time, I resigned from my prestigious job. I was able to continue the practice of medicine, and moved to a small Trust where I now work as a general surgeon, and support with the development of medical students as it is also a teaching hospital.

'My main areas of interest remain predominantly in liver transplant and hepato-pancreato-biliary surgery, though these are now academic interests only, as well as upper gastrointestinal tract and general surgery.

'The most rewarding aspect of my job are the patients. However, the politics that surround medicine at this time are unpleasant. The lack of resources, capacity and at times, the overregulation of our working lives, makes working in the NHS challenging.

'My biggest tip for aspiring doctors is to always be careful of your actions and to protect yourself, as what you may regard as trivial can be taken out of context. You should also ensure that you have a thorough support network, and to make sure that you give yourself a life outside of your career in medicine, as it is easy to be consumed by it.'

Things to consider

The case of Dr Bramhall raised some important concerns and areas of consideration. You might want to think about the following points.

- The patient was entirely unharmed, and it would never have been revealed if it wasn't for unrelated complications.
- Dr Bramhall and several nurses with whom he worked claimed it was merely to relieve tension, reflecting on the working conditions.
- Some people feel that the claims of abuse are extreme, but damage was inflicted on the patient without their consent.
- The patients were in a position of vulnerability as they were under general anaesthetic.
- Irrespective of how trivial an act is, there are significant consequences when it calls into question an abuse of power.

The Charlie Gard case: Great Ormond Street Hospital v Yates and Gard

The Charlie Gard case was an incredibly high profile case in the UK during 2017. It involved Charlie Gard, an infant patient with a rare genetic disorder known as mitochondrial DNA depletion syndrome, which leads to progressive muscle and brain degeneration. Typically, the disease is fatal in infancy because of no available treatment.

The case became controversial as the parents wished to pursue alternative treatment methods, and the medical staff at Great Ormond Street Hospital did not believe that this was in Charlie's best interest.

The case proceeded as follows.

- Charlie was admitted to hospital in October 2016 due to shallow breathing and failure to thrive.
- Charlie was diagnosed with mitochondrial DNA depletion syndrome.
- Dr Hirano, a neurologist from New York, was working on an experimental treatment at the time and was contacted.
- He agreed that they should try the treatment.
- In January 2017, Charlie underwent a series of seizures that caused significant brain damage.
- Great Ormond Street Hospital medical staff determined that further treatment would not be beneficial, and that palliative care should be put in place instead.
- The parents disagreed with this view and raised the funds to transport Charlie to New York for further treatment.
- The High Court supported Great Ormond Street Hospital and overturned the parents' right to take Charlie to New York for further treatment.
- The parents appealed the case to the Court of Appeal, the Supreme Court and the European Court of Human Rights.
- The courts declined these appeals, ruling that it would be in Charlie's best interests to die with dignity.
- Several medical professionals from around the world signed a letter suggesting that controversial and unpublished data showed that the therapy could improve Charlie's condition.
- Great Ormond Street Hospital then called for a new hearing in light of the evidence.
- Dr Hirano flew over from America to assess Charlie's condition and claimed it was too late for the therapy to be effective as Charlie's condition had deteriorated too rapidly.
- Charlie's parents abandoned legal proceedings so that they could cherish the time that they had left with him.
- Charlie was transferred to a hospice and life support was withdrawn.

This was a case that caught the attention of the general public, not only in the UK but around the world. The case was incredibly divisive. Some individuals felt that Charlie should be allowed to die with dignity, rather than causing him further pain through experimental medication. Others felt that his parents had a right to fight for their child's life.

Things to consider

While incredibly sensitive, there were many lessons to be learned from the Charlie Gard case. Things to consider include the following.

- The rights that parents have when considering which actions to take for their child – should the wishes of the parents be overruled by medical professionals?
- Access to experimental medicine – should parents be able to access it if they wish, even in the absence of significant evidence? If a patient is going to die anyway, should it be withheld?
- Even with the treatment, Charlie's condition would not improve, but its progression would slow down. Is it ethical to prolong the life of an individual without cognition and experiencing pain? Is it ethical to not do so?
- Should decisions be made by the courts? Should there be a fairer, faster way of resolving medical disputes?

The Charlie Gard case highlights the complex nature of medical ethics. Ethics is not personal opinion, it is a system of moral principles that demands rational reasoning and careful reflection of individual issues.

Moral and ethical issues

The weighted and complex questions that have a moral and/or ethical dimension constitute a very relevant and current area that has caused large amounts of discussion – and, indeed, can often polarise opinion. Many medical students with whom we have spoken tell us that, almost without exception, either one or several of the following issues were discussed at the interview stage.

When answering questions on ethics, there are no specific answers, and each individual's answer is likely to vary slightly. It is worth applying the four pillars of ethics to your answers to ensure that they are aligned with the core principles of healthcare.

- **Autonomy.** Your actions must respect the rights of the patient, as well as their right to make decisions about their healthcare.
- **Beneficence.** Your actions must be advantageous to the patient.
- **Non-maleficence.** Your actions must not harm the patient.
- **Justice.** You must treat all patients equally.

TIP!

There are several useful documents which you should review when preparing for medical school interviews:

- *Tomorrow's Doctors*, provided by the General Medical Council
- *Medical Ethics Today*, provided by the British Medical Association

Euthanasia and assisted deaths

Euthanasia is illegal in the UK, and doctors alleged to have given a patient a lethal dose of a medication with the intention of ending life will be charged with manslaughter or murder, depending on the circumstances surrounding each case. UK law also prohibits assisting with suicide.

However, in order to prove the offence of aiding and abetting it is necessary to prove firstly that the person in question had taken their own life and, secondly, that an individual or individuals had aided and abetted the person in committing suicide.

In October 2014 the Director of Public Prosecutions (DPP) published an updated policy on prosecuting assisted suicide cases. The Crown Prosecution Service (CPS) website gives details of the public interest factors against prosecution. These include:

1. the victim had reached a voluntary, clear, settled and informed decision to commit suicide
2. the suspect was wholly motivated by compassion
3. the actions of the suspect, although sufficient to come within the definition of the offence, were of only minor encouragement or assistance
4. the suspect had sought to dissuade the victim from taking the course of action which resulted in his or her suicide
5. the actions of the suspect may be characterised as reluctant encouragement or assistance in the face of a determined wish on the part of the victim to commit suicide
6. the suspect reported the victim's suicide to the police and fully assisted them in their enquiries into the circumstances of the suicide or the attempt and his or her part in providing encouragement or assistance.

Source: www.cps.gov.uk/legal-guidance/policy-prosecutors-respect-cases-encouraging-or-assisting-suicide. Contains public sector information licensed under the Open Government Licence v3.0.

The Tony Nicklinson case in March 2012 brought this law into question. Tony Nicklinson was paralysed from the neck down after a stroke, leaving him with 'locked-in syndrome'. While High Court judges sympathised with his case, they refused his appeal to grant immunity to a doctor to help him end his life, stating that it was for Parliament to decide, not the judicial process. Even though Tony Nicklinson died of pneumonia six days after this hearing, having starved himself in response to the verdict, the family continue to fight this ruling for other sufferers in similar predicaments. In 2013, the Court of Appeal rejected cases from Jane Nicklinson and Paul Lamb (who was paralysed after a road accident) despite intervention from the British Humanist Association (BHA), which was seeking to lend its support. A second case was won, however, in a case for a man known only as 'Martin'. A ruling from two Court of Appeal judges said the law should be 'spelt out unambiguously' over whether those seeking to help would be prosecuted, with the DPP now forced to clarify and possibly having to state that prosecutions will not be made against those who aid this decision.

In June 2015, a Bill proposed by Lord Falconer completed its first reading in the House of Lords. If approved by both Houses of Parliament, this new law would have allowed terminally ill, mentally competent adults to request that a doctor provide them with life-ending medication. What is significant is that the doctor would no longer face criminal prosecution for taking a positive step to help end a patient's life. The current law only allows doctors to withdraw medication and sustenance from a patient in a persistent vegetative state.

In 2015, Simon Binner again brought this issue to the media as he posted details of his condition – motor neurone disease – along with the dates of his death and funeral on his LinkedIn page, before flying to Switzerland for assisted suicide, thus continuing to raise the debate about dignity over legality. Following on from Lord Falconer's bill, which simply ran out of time before the General Election, 2015 also saw the Assisted Dying Bill introduced by Rob Marris – the first real move to change UK law on the right to die – which was overwhelmingly rejected by MPs at the second reading, who did not want to make such a controversial change to the law. It is likely that the motion will go before Parliament again in the future as it is an issue which keeps coming up.

You can find more information about the DPP's policy on assisted suicide at www.cps.gov.uk/legal-guidance/suicide-policy-prosecutors-respect-cases-encouraging-or-assisting-suicide.

Things to consider

When answering questions on euthanasia, consider the following.

- Discuss the fact that euthanasia is complex; there are no black and white answers, which makes drawing conclusions difficult.
- Discuss the legal aspects of euthanasia: assisted suicide or active euthanasia is illegal in the UK, but there are other countries where either of these acts, or both of them, are legal. As such, it is worth keeping an eye on any changes in the law.
- Reflect on the ethical considerations: it appeals to the benevolence ethical pillar, yet contrasts with the concept of non-maleficence.
- The ethical guidelines provided by the GMC must ultimately be relied upon.
- Any other factors, such as the mental capacity of the patient and any pressures that may have been applied, must also be rigorously investigated.

Do not fall into the trap of giving your personal opinion, and falling on one side of the argument. It is crucial that you make use of the four pillars of ethics.

Abortion

Even recently there was new controversy regarding abortion, as the BMA issued guidance advising doctors that 'there may be circumstances in which termination of pregnancy on foetal grounds would be lawful'. As reported in the *Telegraph*, there was a backlash from MPs who have criticised the BMA for trying to redefine abortion laws. In the wake of the controversial decision of the CPS not to prosecute two doctors who were secretly filmed offering to abort selected-sex babies, the DPP warned that the guidance for doctors needs urgently to be updated. The current BMA guidance suggests that it is 'unethical' to terminate a pregnancy on the grounds of sex alone, but it also says that the wishes and situation of the mother should be considered. The Law and Ethics of Abortion BMA Views report of November 2014 says that in England, Scotland and Wales, provided the criteria from the Abortion Act 1967 are fulfilled, then abortion is lawful. It goes on to say that unless it is necessary to save the life of the mother, doctors have a right to conscientious objection should they wish.

One in three women will have an abortion before they are 45 years old, and in 2018 there were 200,608 abortions in England and Wales. Yet, without certain conditions being met, abortion is still illegal. Indeed, it has long been the subject of controversy in Northern Ireland, where it was only decriminalised in October 2019.

Things to consider

As with any ethical topic, abortion is a complex area with no clear cut answers. When discussing it, you should consider the following points.

- Outline that it is a controversial issue.
- Discuss the legal aspects – that abortion is legal in the UK up to 24 weeks of pregnancy following the agreement of two doctors that the abortion would be less damaging to the woman's physical and mental health than the pregnancy itself. In rare medical instances, it is legal for abortions to take place after this date.
- When considering the four pillars of ethics, autonomy states that patients have a right to make decisions about their bodies.
- Beneficence suggests that doctors must prioritise the best interests of the patient, which in this case would be the mother, whose mental and physical well-being must be considered.
- Non-maleficence raises possibly the most controversial aspect. While abortion may cause harm to the patient, it also raises questions about the sanctity of human life. On the whole, it is a complex and sensitive element, so regardless of personal opinion, it is best not to dwell on this for too long.
- Again, refer to the ethical guidelines provided by the GMC.

Refusal of treatment

As per the ethical pillar of patient autonomy, patients have the right to make decisions about their own treatment. Before a medical intervention is conducted, patients must give consent, and this is the case for all procedures, ranging from a straightforward blood test to a complex operation.

For a patient to rightfully refuse treatment, the decision must be entirely voluntary, and not a result of coercion by another party, such as a relative or a healthcare professional. In addition, the patient must make the decision in a manner that is informed; they must have a thorough understanding of what the treatment is for, what it entails, possible alternatives and consequences of going through with the refusal.

While patient decisions must be respected, there is an exception to this rule and refusal of treatment can be overturned if the doctor in charge of the patient's care feels that the patient lacks the capacity to make an informed and voluntary decision. In this instance, capacity refers to the ability to demonstrate an understanding of the decision and an ability to communicate it with the healthcare professionals. For the most part, adults are deemed as being capable to make informed and voluntary decisions, but some conditions may influence this, including:

- those with dementia
- those affected by mental health conditions, such as schizophrenia or bipolar disorder
- those under the influence of drugs or alcohol.

Another area of consideration includes advance decisions. Individuals older than 18 years of age can produce what is referred to as a 'living will', which typically details the refusal of medical interventions prior to them being needed, in the case that they might be incapable of making those decisions at the time. One example is the signing of Do Not Attempt Resuscitation (DNAR) forms so that life-saving interventions are not utilised in the case of cardiac arrest.

Things to consider

As with other ethical issues, when discussing refusal of treatment, you must consider all of the ethical arguments associated with the issue.

- Consider the role of the doctor in this situation – they must fully inform the patient of what the treatment is, what it entails, whether there are alternative treatments and the consequences of not accepting the treatment.
- When considering the four pillars of ethics, patient autonomy must be respected.

- The doctor also has a role in assessing the capability of a patient in making the decision, and ensuring that the decision is not being influenced by a third party.
- Beneficence in this situation would be to provide the patient with the treatment that they require.
- However, if this is against the patient's wishes, then it may be that giving the treatment will do more harm than it will good, thereby conflicting with the non-maleficence pillar of ethics.
- Finally, refer to the GMC's guidelines on the situation.

Other ethical questions

The ethical considerations in medicine are extensive, and you should research as many as possible. As a starting point, you should consider some of the following points.

- A patient is diagnosed with Huntington's disease, but does not want to pass the information on to his children, from whom he is estranged.
- The importance of patient confidentiality when dealing with a child.
- The NHS should not fund treatment for diseases that are a result of obesity.
- You witness a colleague upsetting a patient by being rude and offensive.
- You are working as a doctor and your colleague and friend, also a practising doctor, turns up to work under the influence of alcohol.
- You have two patients who require a liver transplant and a liver becomes available that suits both of them. One is an ex-alcoholic mother with two young children while the other is a teenager who was born with a liver defect. Who do you give it to?

Remember, not all ethical scenarios will be directly related to medicine. They may ask you about something entirely unrelated to assess your reaction, so don't be surprised if this happens at interview!

8 | Results day

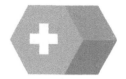

The A level results will arrive at your school on the third Thursday in August. For International Baccalaureate (IB) qualifications results day will be in the first week of July and for students studying in Scotland it will be the first week of August. The medical schools will have received them a few days earlier. You must make sure that you are at home on the day the results are published and able to travel in to your school or college to collect them. If you are unable to do this, speak to your school or college about making arrangements for your results to be given to you by phone or email as early as possible on the day; don't wait for the school to post the results slip to you. If you need to act to secure a place, you may have to do so quickly. This chapter will take you through the steps you should take after receiving your results and also explains what to do if your grades are below what you expected.

If things go wrong during the exams

If something happens when you are preparing for or actually taking the exams that prevents you from doing your best, you must notify your school/college, who should then notify the exam board and the medical schools that have made you offers. Ensure that these parties are made aware of your stuation as soon as possible; it is no good waiting for disappointing results and then telling everyone that you felt ghastly at the time but said nothing to anyone. Exam boards can give you special consideration if the appropriate forms are sent to them by the school, along with supporting evidence. An increasing number of medical schools now only accept mitigating circumstances if they were reported to the exam board at the time of the examination.

Your extenuating circumstances must be significant. A 'slight sniffle' won't do! If you really are sufficiently ill to be unable to prepare for the exams or to perform effectively during them, you must consult your GP and obtain a letter describing your condition.

The other main cause of underperformance is distressing events at home. If a member of your immediate family is very seriously ill, or if you have some form of significant domestic upheaval, you should explain this to your head teacher and ask him or her to write to the examiners and medical schools.

With luck, the medical schools may allow you to slip one grade below the conditional offer, although this is rare and should not be relied upon. If things work out badly, then the fact that you declared extenuating circumstances should ensure that you are treated sympathetically if you decide to reapply through UCAS.

The medical school admissions departments are well organised and efficient, but they are staffed by human beings. If there were extenuating circumstances that could have affected your exam performance and that were brought to their notice in June, it is a good idea to ask them to review the relevant letters shortly before the exam results are published.

If you hold an offer and get the grades

If you previously received a conditional offer and your grades equal or exceed that offer, congratulations! You can relax and wait for your chosen medical school to send you joining instructions. One word of warning: you cannot assume that grades of A*AB satisfy an AAA offer. This is especially true if the B grade is in biology or chemistry. You should call your chosen university as soon as possible to check if you have met your offer.

If you have good grades but no offer

Very few schools keep places open and, of those that do, most will choose to allow applicants who hold a conditional offer to slip a grade rather than dust off a reserve list of those they interviewed but didn't make an offer to. They are even less likely to consider applicants who appear out of the blue, no matter how high their grades are. In recent years, a small number of universities have offered Clearing places. With the increased number of places being made available for studying medicine at university, it is possible that more spaces will be available through Clearing, although this is not an option that should be relied upon.

If you hold three A grades but were rejected when you applied through UCAS, you need to let the medical schools know that you are out there. The best way to do this is by phone and email. Places available to students in this position are few and far between, so it is preferable to phone in order to make contact as quickly as possible. Contact details are listed in the UCAS directory and are on the university websites.

Set out below is sample text for an email, which can also be used as the basis of a phone call. Make sure you write your own version of this; don't copy it word for word!

To: Mrs Lister

Subject: Application to study medicine at Rushmere University

Dear Mrs Lister

UCAS no. 16-024680-8

I applied to study medicine at Rushmere University this year. I regrettably was rejected as a result of my interview/without an interview, which at the time I was disappointed to hear. Today I received grades:

Biology – A
Chemistry – A*
Maths – A*

While I appreciate this is a very busy time of year for you and that it is non-standard to take applicants at this stage of the year, I am contacting you to see if, after results day, there were any places still at Rushmere University to study medicine. I learned a great deal from my interview experience previously and I would be very willing to attend another interview at short notice to demonstrate that I have taken on board the advice I was given.

I look forward to hearing from you.

Yours sincerely,

Charlotte Stevenson

If, despite your most strenuous efforts, you are unsuccessful, you need to consider applying again (see below). The other alternative is to use the Clearing system to obtain a place on a degree course related to medicine and prepare to apply again once you have completed your first degree.

UCAS Adjustment process

The UCAS Adjustment option is for students who have accepted an offer of a place and then achieve higher grades. A typical case might be the student who accepts a CCC offer to study bioengineering and then achieves AAA. He or she then has a short period of time (usually a week) to register for Adjustment in order to be able to approach universities that require higher grades.

It is unlikely that potential medics would be able to gain places this way, since there are very few medical places available in the post-results period and those that are available would normally be allocated to students who applied for medicine in the first place. But if you are in this situation, there is nothing to be lost by contacting the medical schools to see if they can consider you. Contact details for each university can be found on the UCAS website.

If you hold an offer but miss the grades

If you have only narrowly missed the required grades, you can contact the medical school to put your case forward. Most universities will have made their decision in advance of results day and are unlikely to be swayed; however, there is nothing to be lost by trying. Sample text for another email follows below.

To: Mrs Lister

Subject: Application to study medicine at Rushmere University

Dear Mrs Lister

UCAS no. 16-024680-8

I have a place to study medicine at Rushmere University this year. However, I am afraid that having received my results, I found that I have missed my offer. Today I received grades:

Biology – B
Chemistry – A
Maths – A*

As you can see, I just missed my offer by one grade in Biology, though I received a higher grade than anticipated in Maths. Therefore, I was wondering if you could guide me as to whether my grades are still applicable for my place or what the next steps are if my place is to be rescinded.

I look forward to hearing from you and remain resolute and determined to achieve my place at Rushmere University, as for me, it is without question where I wish to develop and train as a doctor.

Yours sincerely,

Charlotte Stevenson

If this is unsuccessful, you need to consider retaking your A levels and applying again (see below). The other alternative is to use the Clearing system to try and obtain a place on a degree course related to medicine and prepare to apply to a medical course after you graduate.

Retaking A levels

The grade requirements for retake candidates are potentially higher than for first-timers (usually A*AA). You should retake any subject where your first result was below B and you should aim for at least an A grade.

Remember that if you resit A levels under the current system, you have to take all of the exams again, with no guarantee that your grade will improve. So if you already have a B grade and then secure a C grade in your resit year, the C grade will stand.

Check with your college or school on its provisions for students wanting to retake. It is also possible to retake A levels at some further education and independent colleges. Interviews to discuss this are free and carry no obligation to enrol on a course, so it is worth taking the time to talk to their staff before you embark on A level retakes.

It is possible to resit IB examinations. This is available in either November or May, though you would have to complete within three opportunities to complete the qualification. You can retake a Scottish Higher in a separate academic year and the same is true for Advanced Highers, but not in all subjects. You would have to register again for, and then resit, the Advanced Highers. The same applies for the IB examinations, as you would effectively need to sit the whole qualification again.

Reapplying to medical school

Many medical schools discourage retake candidates (see Table 11, pages 221–224), so the whole business of applying again needs careful thought, hard work and a bit of luck. The choice of medical schools for your UCAS application will be narrower than it was the first time round, so it is vital to carefully research which universities you will be eligible to apply to. Don't apply to the medical schools that discourage retakers unless there really are special, extenuating circumstances to explain your disappointing grades, such as:

- your own illness
- the death or serious illness of a very close relative
- serious domestic upheaval, such as divorce.

These are just guidelines; the only safe method of finding out if a medical school will accept you is to ask directly. Send an email so that you can have a record of the reply that they send. Text for a typical email is set out below. Don't follow it slavishly and do take the time to write to a wide range of medical schools before you make your final choice.

To: Mrs Lister

Subject: Application to study medicine at Rushmere University

Dear Mrs Lister

UCAS no. 16-024680-8

I am hopeful of applying to Rushmere University this year but I am retaking my A levels.

This year, I received the following grades

Biology – B
Chemistry – B
Spanish – B

I am retaking all of the above and am expected to achieve at least A grades in all subjects.

I note that you encourage retake applicants in specific circumstances; however, I am not sure if I would be eligible and I hope that you will be able to advise me. I do not have any extenuating circumstances that have affected my performance.

I look forward to hearing from you.

Yours sincerely,

Charlotte Stevenson

Notice that the format of your email should be:

- opening paragraph
- your exam results: set out clearly and with no omissions
- any extenuating circumstances: a brief statement
- your retake plan, including the timescale
- a request for help and advice
- closing formalities.

Make sure that it is brief, clear and well presented. Apart from the care needed in making the choice of medical school, the rest of the application procedure is as described in the first section of this book.

The same advice applies if you are reapplying with qualifications other than A levels. If you did not get a place but now have the grades required, then you will probably be able to reapply, but make sure you talk to the medical schools first. If you have not got the grades, then you need to look at what routes are available. If you do not resit the IB, you will need to look at A levels or Foundation programmes in order to reach the requisite entry requirements for a medicine course. If you have taken Scottish Highers, depending on the subject, you are able to retake again in a new academic year. Either way, you must make sure that you gain the necessary qualifications in the next sitting – even though this will allow entry to only a handful of medical schools, you should still make contact and speak to the admissions tutors at those medical schools that consider retakes.

Case study

Pranay is a second-year medical student at King's College, London. After underachieving in his first attempt at A levels, Pranay secured his offer while retaking Biology, Chemistry and Mathematics, in which he achieved grades A*A*A respectively.

'I chose to study medicine as it is a dynamic and rapidly advancing profession that enables me to gain an understanding of the human body in immense depth and then apply that knowledge to patients in order to improve their quality of life as best as possible. Additionally, medicine is multi-faceted and with a huge range of clinical specialities, along with research and teaching opportunities. I will be constantly learning and bettering myself as a doctor as my career progresses.

'Unfortunately, when I took my A levels for the first time, I did not achieve the grades I wanted. However, I always knew that studying medicine was my goal, so I decided to undertake a one-year A level programme at an independent sixth-form college in Birmingham, where I received huge support and guidance and as a result I was able to achieve A*A*A and take up a place to study medicine at King's College, London.

'I've really enjoyed the course so far. It is intense and demanding, but the content is stimulating and there are a variety of teaching methods, including lectures, tutorials, workshops, laboratory practicals and dissections. In Year 1, dissections were particularly enjoyable as you get hands on experience with a cadaver – a captivating way to learn anatomy, although you never get used to the smell!

'The workload is intensive and requires you to be very well organised to stay on top of it all – but this is a skill that you'll need throughout life as a doctor so is actually very beneficial.

'I found that Year 1 was a bombardment of scientific knowledge through the medium of lectures, tutorials and workshops, with very little chance to develop clinical skills. However, in Year 2 we will start general practice and hospital placements, which provides the chance to apply our knowledge to real clinical scenarios.

'The process of applying to medicine can be very daunting, but I would say focus on each step at a time, whether that be the UCAT or BMAT, your personal statement, your interviews or gaining relevant work experience. Try not to overwhelm yourself, because as you overcome each step, the next one tends to fall into place.

'Also, make sure that you are prepared for the interviews, especially the MMI format that most medical schools use nowadays. I used a lot of live examples from my work experience and personal life that was aligned to the skill of a doctor at all my interviews. At interviews, be yourself and let your personality shine. The application and selection process is pretty time consuming, so ensure you allocate enough time for it. When selecting medical schools, I found it very informative to talk to the admissions tutors about my application and their interview process. For example, King's College said their primary selection criteria for interview was a 700+ UCAT score, while Cardiff wanted 8 A* GCSE grades, so each university was unique; and admissions tutors were always very open as to whether I had a strong application or not.

'Constantly remind yourself why you want to be a doctor and use that drive as motivation to work hard and be organised as these skills will benefit you greatly during your time at medical school.

'Lastly, do things you enjoy and have fun; don't do loads of different activities just to put it on your personal statement if you don't find them fulfilling. If you commit to activities you enjoy, that passion will come across if you're asked about it at interview!'

9 | Non-standard applications

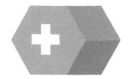

So far, this book has been concerned with the 'standard' applicant: the UK resident who is studying at least two science subjects at A level/ in the IB course/Scottish Highers – and who is applying from school or who is retaking immediately after disappointing grades. However, what about students who do not have this 'standard' background, such as international students? Or those who have not studied science A levels? The main non-standard applicants and the steps they should take to apply to medical school are outlined in this chapter.

Those who have not studied science A levels

If you decide that you would like to study medicine after having already started on a combination of A levels that does not fit the subject requirements for entry to medical school, you are potentially eligible to apply for the 'pre-medical course'.

The course covers elements of chemistry, biology and physics and prepares you for the demands of the degree course. The pre-medical course lasts one academic year. If your application is rejected, you will have to spend a further two years taking science A levels at a sixth-form college. Alternatively, some colleges offer one-year A level courses, and many subjects can be covered from scratch in a single year. However, only very able students can cover A levels in chemistry and biology in a single year with good results. You should discuss your particular circumstances with the staff of a number of colleges in order to select the course that will prepare you to achieve the A level grades you need in the subjects you require.

Overseas students

Competition for the few places available to overseas students is fierce, and you would be wise to discuss your application informally with the medical school before submitting your UCAS application. The UCAS website gives a useful overview of international student statistics that illustrate perfectly the difficulties faced by international applicants. For example, in 2019, there were a total of 80,995 applications for medicine, with 63,175 from domestic students, 5,900 from EU students and 11,925 from non-EU international students. Some 8,465 domestic students, 310 EU students and 875 non-EU international students were accepted.

Many medical schools give preference to students who do not have adequate provision for training in their own countries. You should contact the medical schools individually for advice on the application procedure and costs.

Following the UK's departure from the EU in January 2020 and the end of the transition period in January 2021, it is now clear that EU students will be treated in a similar way to non-EU international students in the future, particularly in terms of the fees they pay. This is most likely to lead to a reduction of EU applicants, but paradoxically may cause the number of EU students admitted to study medicine to increase due to the more lucrative fee levels that may be charged by the universities.

At the time of writing, the government has stated that EU students starting study on or after 1 August 2021 will not be eligible for home fee status or financial support from Student Finance unless they are normally resident in the UK. Further details can be found at www.gov.uk/guidance/studying-in-the-uk-guidance-for-eu-students.

Mature students and graduates

Graduates

Course options available to graduates include the following:

- four-year graduate-entry courses
- five-year courses in the normal way
- some six-year pre-medical/medical courses
- Access to Medicine Diploma courses.

You should check which Access to Medicine Diploma courses are accepted by medical schools, as many will not consider them. Often, each medical school has a shortlist of Access courses from which it accepts applications – for example, at Keele they currently look only at the Access course from Bolton College, College of West Anglia (CWA), Dudley College, Harlow College, Truro and Penwith College, Manchester College, Stafford College and Sussex Downs College. It is also usually the case that you have to reach a very high level of achievement in these courses, not just pass them.

Mature students

In recent years the options available for mature students have increased enormously. There is a growing awareness that older students often represent a 'safer' option for medical schools because they are likely to be more committed to medicine and less likely to drop out, and are able to bring to the medical world many skills and experiences that 18-year-olds sometimes lack. In general, there are two types of mature applicant:

1. those who have always wanted to study medicine but who failed to get into medical school when they applied from school in the normal way
2. those who came to the idea later on in life, often having embarked on a totally different career.

The first type of mature applicant has usually followed a degree course in a subject related to medicine and has obtained a good grade (minimum 2.i). This pathway is well trodden and there are many medical professionals who have entered the profession via this route. The second category of mature student is those who have achieved success in other careers and who can bring a breadth of experience to the medical school and to the profession.

Options available for mature students are summarised below. The chapter then examines each option in more detail.

Applicants with A levels that satisfy medical schools' standard offers
Can apply for five-/six-year courses in the normal way.

Applicants with A levels that do not satisfy standard offers
This could include arts A levels, or grades that are too low. Applicants in this category can take the following routes.

- Retake/pick up new A levels at sixth-form college and apply for five-/six-year courses in the normal way.
- Enrol on a six-year course that includes a preliminary year. These courses are designed for students who achieved high grades at A level but did not take the required number of science subjects to apply for the A100 course. The courses are available at:
  o Cardiff
  o Liverpool
  o Manchester
  These courses include a foundation (pre-medical) year and are designed for students without science A level backgrounds, although the exact combination of permitted A level subjects varies between universities. They should not be confused with the six-year (usually A100) courses offered by many medical schools that include an intercalated BSc.
- Enrol on a six-year course that includes a gateway year. These courses are designed for able students who have specific contextual factors that have impacted on their attainment and fulfil specific widening participation criteria. Before considering applying to one of

these courses, you must carefully investigate their criteria to ensure that you are eligible. The courses are available at:

- o Aberdeen
- o Bristol
- o Bradford
- o Dundee
- o Edge Hill
- o UEA
- o Glasgow
- o Hull York
- o King's
- o Lancaster
- o Leeds
- o Leicester
- o Lincoln
- o Liverpool
- o Nottingham
- o Plymouth
- o Southampton
- o St Andrews
- Enrol on an Access course (see page 187).

Mature students with no formal A level or equivalent qualifications

Applicants in this category can take the following routes:

- A levels, then five-/six-year courses in the normal way
- Access courses (see page 187).

Preparing the application

Mature students and graduates are faced with many decisions on the route to becoming a doctor. Not only do they have to decide which course or combination of courses might be suitable, but in many cases they also have to try to gauge how best to juggle the conflicting demands of study, financial practicalities and their families.

Mature students need to prepare carefully for their applications in order to ensure that they are recognised as being fully committed to a career as a doctor. Typically, when a mature student is interviewed, the interviewers are interested in:

- why you have decided to change direction
- what you have done to convince yourself that this is the right career path
- what your career has given you in the way of personal qualities that are relevant to medicine
- what skills and personal qualities you have developed in your previous career that are relevant to medicine.

Case study

Erzsike is currently working as a Foundation Year 1 doctor after studying on the graduate-entry programme at the University of Birmingham. Though this was not her initial plan, she is appreciative of the route that she took, as studying an undergraduate degree allowed her to develop the skills required to succeed in the study of medicine.

'My pathway into medicine was slightly longer than most students. While completing the IB, my application to study medicine was unsuccessful, so I opted to complete a BMedSci undergraduate degree at the University of Birmingham, which took three years to complete. Following this, I worked as a healthcare assistant for a year and reapplied for Graduate Entry Medicine at the University of Birmingham. Throughout the process of applying, I had to cope with rejection a number of times, but I feel that my pathway into medicine has ultimately given me a greater range of skills compared to if I had entered as an 18-year-old.

'I currently work in a hospital in Birmingham as a Foundation Year 1 doctor in General Medicine. It took me a while to get used to the long hours that I had to work and the busy on-call shifts, but these things get easier with time. In spite of the difficult elements of the job, the changes I can make to people's care each day make it all worthwhile.

'In the future, I am aiming to become a GP with a specialist interest in palliative care, an area of medicine that truly focuses on patients as a whole and their quality of life.

'At this point in time, I feel that the current hot topics in the world of medicine include mental health, e-cigarettes and the rise of preventable conditions such as cardiovascular disease and diabetes.

'My advice for aspiring medics is to consider your personal and unique reasons for your interest in medicine and link these to the qualities mentioned in GMC's "Tomorrow's Doctors" document in order to really "build a picture" of yourself on paper in your personal statement. It is also important to gain a genuine insight into the career through work experience and volunteering in order to gain the skills for a lifetime of working with people.'

Personal statement

When writing your personal statement, try to get a number of people to read it and give you their opinion. However, the most useful opinions will come from academic staff at your school or college or doctors who have a role in recruiting students. Keep your writing simple, make sure to write in continuous prose, don't overuse the thesaurus, and check spelling and punctuation extremely carefully. Remember, spell check isn't foolproof and won't flag the difference between 'principle' and 'principal', or 'effect' and 'affect'. It's the little things like that which undermine a perfectly good application.

For mature applicants, the UCAS personal statement needs to be carefully structured. The strictly limited space means that a convincing case has to be constructed in a concise manner.

For mature applicants, the personal statement should be structured as follows.

1. Why you want to study medicine.
2. Brief career and educational history.
3. Reasons for the change of direction.
4. What you have done to investigate medicine, including work experience and voluntary work.
5. Brief details of achievements, interests.

The most important thing to bear in mind is that you must convince the selectors that you are serious about the change in direction, and that your decision to apply to study medicine is not a spur-of-the-moment reaction to dissatisfaction with your current job or studies.

A useful exercise is to try to imagine that you are the person who will read the personal statement in order to decide whether to interview or to reject without interview. Does your personal statement contain sufficient indication of thorough research, preparation and long-term commitment? If it does not, you will be rejected. As a rough guide, approximately three-quarters of it should cover your reasons for applying for a medical course and the preparation and research that you have undertaken. The further back in time you can demonstrate that you started to plan your application, the stronger it will be.

Applying for a Gateway course

Gateway courses or programmes are not to be confused with Access courses. As the name suggests, these courses usually act as a 'gateway' for entering Year 1 of a standard medical course.

You will need to look at the website of each medical university to find out if it offers this course. These courses are now specifically aimed at widening participation of students from deprived backgrounds and so are not appropriate for all students. Make sure you look carefully at the eligibility details to ensure that you meet the criteria for any course you are considering applying to.

Access courses

A number of colleges of further education offer Access to Medicine courses. The best-known and most successful of these is the course at the College of West Anglia, in King's Lynn. Primarily (but not exclusively) aimed at health professionals, such as nurses and paramedics, the course covers biology, chemistry, physics and other medically related topics, and lasts one year. Some medical schools will accept students who have successfully completed the course, but it is important to check which universities you will be able to apply to before commencing. Contact details can be found at the end of the book.

Four-year graduate courses

Often known as Graduate Entry Programmes (GEPs), these are usually given the code A101 or A102 by UCAS. The first medical schools to introduce accelerated courses specifically for graduates were St George's Hospital Medical School and Leicester/Warwick (which has since split into two separate medical schools). Courses can be divided into two types:

1. those for graduates with a medically related degree
2. those that accept graduates with degrees in any discipline.

The following medical schools run GEPs, further details of which can be found on the UCAS website:

- Birmingham
- Cambridge
- Cardiff
- Dundee and St Andrews (ScotGEM)
- King's
- Liverpool
- Newcastle
- Nottingham
- Oxford
- Queen Mary
- Sheffield
- Southampton
- St George's
- Swansea
- Warwick.

Graduate pre-admissions tests

The BMAT and UCAT are used by some graduate-entry providers. Alongside this, six programmes use the GAMSAT (Graduate Medical School Admissions Test). The universities using each test are summarised in Table 8, see page 188.

Standard registrations for the GAMSAT UK test take place in mid-May for those sitting the test in September, and in early November for those sitting the test in March. The fee to sit the GAMSAT test is £268, but an extra charge of £60 applies if you register for the GAMSAT after the main closing date. Payment must be made by credit card at the time of completing your online registration. Candidates sit the GAMSAT examination in either March or September, and those with the best all-round scores are then called for interview. The GAMSAT examination consists of three papers, which are all taken on the same day.

1. Reasoning in humanities and social sciences (47 multiple-choice questions) – 70 minutes, including 6 minutes' reading time.
2. Written communication (two writing tasks) – 65 minutes, including 5 minutes' reading time.
3. Reasoning in biological and physical sciences (75 multiple-choice questions: 40% biology, 40% chemistry, 20% physics) – 150 minutes, including 8 minutes' reading time.

The GAMSAT website (https://gamsat.acer.org/) contains full details of the test along with practice test materials. This is a far more significant test than the UCAT or BMAT and, as such, it would be expected that more time is spent in preparation for it than either of the other two.

Table 8 Graduate-entry medicine courses and their required admissions test

University	Pre-admissions test
Birmingham	UCAT
Cambridge	None
Cardiff	GAMSAT
King's	UCAT
Liverpool	GAMSAT
Newcastle	UCAT
Nottingham	GAMSAT
Oxford	BMAT
Queen Mary	UCAT
ScotGEM	GAMSAT
Sheffield	UCAT
Southampton	UCAT
St George's	GAMSAT
Swansea	GAMSAT
Warwick	UCAT

Private universities

At the University of Buckingham, the first private medical school in the UK opened in January 2015. It currently costs £37,500 per year and will fast-track medical students in four-and-a-half years rather than the standard five or six years. The university is hoping to attract students who would otherwise have looked to study abroad and, as such, is potentially of interest to mature students.

Studying outside the UK

If you are unsuccessful in gaining a place at a UK medical school, and do not want to follow the graduate-entry path, you might want to look at other options. Note that following the UK's decision to leave the EU, arrangements for UK students studying at institutions in other EU countries have changed. If you wish to study a whole degree course in an EU member state after 31 December 2020, it is likely that you will pay a different level of fees which will be based on international student fees.

One option for those who have been unsuccessful with their applications is to study medicine abroad – for example at Charles University in the Czech Republic or Comenius University in Bratislava, the capital of Slovakia. There are a number of medical schools throughout the world that will accept A level students, but the important issue is whether or not you would be able to practise in the UK upon qualification, should you wish to do so. You need to bear in mind that there is a big difference between European and non-European medical schools. In the case of medical schools based within the EU, they are usually fully recognised by the GMC under current European legislation for primary qualifications.

However, one should be cautious with those based in Eastern Europe as statistics show that they often have an alarmingly high drop-out rate. They usually admit students based on a short written entrance test based in science and not always based on a traditional A level syllabus that you may have prepared for. They also do not put much emphasis on your actual A level grades, which does mean that sometimes the wrong students are admitted, which may be a factor in their high attrition rate. Please do your research and be cautious, as often it is staying in medical school that tends to be the challenge, *not* getting in.

In the EU, in addition to the ones mentioned above, you will find examples of such medical schools as Plovdiv Medical University, Bulgaria, Masaryk University, Czech Republic, Palacky University, Czech Republic, Università degli Studi di Milano, Italy, Riga Stradins University, Latvia and Lithuania University of Health Sciences, Lithuania.

There are a wide range of courses outside of the EU attended by UK students. To then practise in the UK, students must sit the PLAB (Professional and Linguistic Assessment Board) test before applying for registration (www.gmc-uk.org/registration-and-licensing/join-the-register/plab). An example of a well-known non-EU course is St George's University School of Medicine in Grenada. Students who wish to practise in the UK can spend part of the clinical stage of the course in a range of hospitals in the UK. Clinical experience can also be gained in hospitals in the US, allowing students to practise there as well. A high proportion of the St George's University medical school teachers have worked in UK universities and medical schools.

In addition to the medical schools attached to UK universities, there are a number of institutions offering medical degree courses that are taught in the UK but are accredited by overseas universities – mostly based in the Caribbean, Russia or Africa. If you are considering these, you must ensure that you are fully satisfied that the courses are bona fide and that the qualification you receive will allow you to practise in the UK (or anywhere else in the world).

In order to check if your qualification is recognised in the UK, you should visit the GMC website (www.gmc-uk.org/registration-and-licensing/join-the-register/before-you-apply/acceptable-overseas-qualifications). You can also refer to the university websites, which should inform you of the validity of their degree in the UK.

Studying abroad may not be the first choice for students who were initially hoping to secure a place at home in the UK. Also, healthcare systems outside the UK are very different, so adapting to life abroad where the local language may not be English as well as studying medicine may not appeal to all.

Case study

After completing an undergraduate degree in the UK, Vinay opted to study at a European university to complete his medicine degree. He is now in his fifth year and has been able to reflect on the pros and cons of studying abroad.

'After the third attempt of failing to get into a medical school in the UK, in spite of me gaining four A grades at A level, I applied to study abroad. I extensively researched the different European universities online for the best university for me to study medicine in English. I chose to apply to the Medical University of Plovdiv in Bulgaria and I am currently in my fifth year of study.

'My experience of studying abroad has been a positive one overall and there are some major advantages compared to studying in the UK. Firstly, the cost of living and studying is much lower; tuition fees, food and accommodation are all much cheaper and student loans are available from the Bulgarian banks. The weather is great and the people are really friendly.

'On the negative side, the teaching standards and overall quality of the university are not as high as in the UK. There are also differences in how the system works in Bulgaria compared to the UK and this can be difficult to get used to. Also the language barrier can be difficult to overcome. However, I am really enjoying my experience and have really liked studying here.'

Getting into US medical schools

While it is possible for international students to study medicine in the United States, it certainly is not straightforward. Firstly, you should go to the AAMC (Association of American Medical Colleges) website at www.aamc.org. This is an excellent site, but can be difficult to navigate to find the information you need. All of the member universities are listed, and by following the links most of your questions can be answered.

Furthermore, from here you can be directed to AMCAS, which is the American Medical College Application Service. For students wishing to apply, go to https://students-residents.aamc.org/applying-medical-school/applying-medical-school-process/applying-medical-school-amcas. The fee is $170 for an application to one school and $40 for every school applied to thereafter. The AAMC website suggests that a very good investment is the *Medical School Admission Requirements (MSAR)*, which can be bought as an online resource for around $28 from https://store.aamc.org.

In the US, medicine is a postgraduate degree. All medical students have completed four years of a science-based or pre-med undergraduate course. You are also expected to gain work experience in these first two years. For more information go to https://students-residents.aamc.org/choosing-medical-career/medical-careers/aspiring-docs.

Suffice to say that the following criteria have to be met.

- Very high grades in A levels – nearly all straight A grades. The higher the grades, the higher your GPA (grade point average) will be; the higher your GPA, the better your chances of being selected by the more renowned universities. An A grade = 4 GPA points; a B grade = 3 points; and a C = 2 points.
- At least one year of biology, physics and English and two years of chemistry (including organic chemistry) post-16/at A level.
- A first degree in a science subject.
- Two or three references from your personal tutor and teachers.
- If you are not from an English-speaking country you will be required to sit the TOEFL (Test of English as a Foreign Language). The minimum score for entry into any university is 79 out of 120. The more demanding the course (such as medicine) and the more prestigious the university, the higher this language requirement will be. Most universities accept the IELTS (International English Language Testing System), but it must be at 7 points or above. The TOEFL test can be sat in the UK.

If you are serious about applying, you need to start as early as possible – early in the first year of your undergraduate programme is recommended. This is because you will need to research the universities as best you can, bearing in mind that the distance does not allow for quick visits to open days as for UK universities. It is also important to remember that fees and living costs are very high; a list of fees and costs can be obtained from the AAMC website.

MCAT

Almost every medical school in the US and Canada requires students to take this 7.5-hour examination. It is a computer-based, multiple-choice assessment, which is divided into four sections.

1. Chemical and Physical Foundations of Biological Systems.
2. Biological and Biochemical Foundations of Living Systems.
3. Psychological, Social, and Biological Foundations of Behaviour.
4. Critical Analysis and Reasoning Skills.

This exam is to be taken in the year that you intend to start study. You can take it up to three times in a year, or four times over two years and a maximum of seven times in total in any number of years. Test dates tend to generally be spread between January and September each year, and you are recommended to register at least 60 days beforehand to ensure that you get a space. It costs $320.

Visas

If you are studying outside the EU, you will require a visa for study. The university in question will advise you on which visa you should obtain; for example, in the USA they will advise you as to whether you require an F-1 Student visa. You do not require a student visa for Grenada if you have a valid British passport. A good place to look first would be the website for the US embassy in the UK at https://uk.usembassy.gov/visas/study-exchange/student. Arrangements for UK citizens for rights of movement within Europe have recently changed due to Brexit. From January 2021, you may need a visa or permit to stay longer than 90 days in a 180-day period. It is essential to research the requirements of each individual country by visiting their embassy website.

Students with disabilities and special educational needs

If a candidate has a specific health requirement or disability there is every possibility that a medical school will be able to help. There is an area in the personal details section of the UCAS application where you can indicate the type of disability/special needs that you have. You need to select the most appropriate option from the list given. There is also a space provided for you to give any further details of the conditions that affect you.

However, each medical school has a responsibility to ensure that doctors are able to fulfil their responsibilities. The decision on fitness to practise is separate from the academic and non-academic selection process. These guidelines are set out by the GMC. You are encouraged to fully research the demands of the course before you apply to each institution. The profession places huge demands on the individual and therefore you must consider all the facts from the outset.

You are equally encouraged to apply if you have a hearing or visual impairment. All institutions are fully committed to support students with special needs, from dyslexia to physical disability, and have access arrangements in place.

Once an offer is made, the medical school will contact you to discuss any appropriate arrangements that should be made. It is most likely to be the case that certain halls of residence may have physical limitations on access arrangements. It is absolutely vital that all relevant information that may impair your ability to study and potentially practise is made clear at this stage. If not, and if the issues become obvious later on in the course, it could possibly result in the candidate being withdrawn from the course.

In terms of special educational needs, students who require a word processor or extra time will be allowed these in the same way that they would have been at school, subject to providing the correct documentation to the university. For more information refer directly to the university.

Some useful websites

Access-Ability: www.accessability.org.uk
Health Careers: www.healthcareers.nhs.uk/explore-roles/doctors/career-opportunities-doctors/doctors-disabilities
GMC: www.gmc-uk.org/education/standards-guidance-and-curricula/guidance/welcomed-and-valued/disabled-doctors-exist

10 | Fees and funding

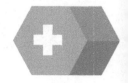

Whether undertaking an undergraduate or postgraduate course, the cost of studying is considerable. This has been exacerbated in recent years by rises in living costs and the large increases in university tuition fees following the publication of the Browne review in 2010. A 2018 study carried out by the British Medical Association (www.bma.org.uk) calculated that average debt among the respondents was £43,700, with values ranging from £600 to £210,500. This overall cost to students will fluctuate depending on a number of factors, some of which are listed below.

- Geographical location: studying in London is going to be more expensive than studying in Birmingham, for example.
- Area of permanent residence: there are differences in fees payable and help available depending on the region of the UK you are from.
- Parental help: contributions from parents may significantly help meet the cost of living.
- Availability of scholarships for exceptional students.
- Paid part-time work, although it has the potential to interfere with your studies.

When considering levels of student debt, it is easy to become disheartened and think that university study is not for you. What all students must remember is that tuition fees do not have to be paid up front; in fact, most students receive student loans to cover this cost. In addition, the loans do not start to be paid back until you are earning over a certain amount (see page 197).

Undertaking a course such as medicine should only be done after seriously considering the overall cost and carefully examining your ability to be fully committed to your study for the full five years. Carefully plan your finances in advance so that you are prepared to cover the cost of tuition fees, living expenses, books and other necessary equipment. Remember, living costs in big cities such as London will be much higher than in other parts of the country.

To find out what the fees are and what funding is available for medical courses, you should explore each of the universities' websites and/or talk to their financial departments, because fees and funding procedures vary from university to university. However, due to the high quality of education provided by medical schools, it is usual for them to charge the maximum level of fees permitted.

Fees

UK students

UK nationals pay lower tuition fees than international students. From September 2018, universities have been able to charge up to the maximum tuition fees of £9,250 per year; it is expected that this figure will rise in line with inflation in the future. The rise in fees is part of the government's Teaching Excellence Framework (TEF), which assesses universities and colleges on the quality of their teaching. The institutions with a TEF award will be able to charge the maximum amount of £9,250, whereas those without a TEF award will only be able to charge £9,000. Tuition fee loans will also increase to cover the higher fees. The fee cap for students studying in Wales remains at £9,000, while fees for students in Northern Ireland are a maximum of £9,250.

There are a number of differences between the systems in England, Scotland, Wales and Northern Ireland, which can result in significant differences between the fees that are ultimately paid by students. From September 2018, the rules are as follows, although they may be subject to change in the future.

- English students are liable for the full fees being charged regardless of where they study within the UK, although for Welsh universities, the maximum amount being charged is still £9,000.
- Students living in Scotland who wish to study full time at a Scottish university are not required to pay tuition fees as long as eligibility criteria are met. Scottish students who wish to study at a university in England or Northern Ireland are required to pay fees of up to £9,250 per academic year. If studying in Wales, fees of up to £9,000 per academic year will be payable.
- For students residing in Wales, up to £9,250 per academic year will be payable if studying at an English, Scottish or Northern Irish university. Welsh students wanting to study in Wales will pay £9,000 per year.
- Students living in Northern Ireland who wish to study in Northern Ireland will pay £4,395 per academic year. Northern Irish students who wish to study elsewhere in the UK are required to pay up to £9,250 per academic year for studying in England or Scotland and £9,000 for studying in Wales.

EU students

Historically, EU students wishing to study in the UK have been eligible to pay the same level of fees as home students. However, this will change significantly for students starting courses after August 2021 due to the completion of the Brexit process. EU students that start studying in the UK after this point will pay an 'EU fee', which will be set by each university. It is likely that the level of fees will be equivalent to the fees charged to international students from outside of the EU. Students from the EU will also lose their entitlement to receive student loans from the government to fund their study in the UK. At this point, it appears that students from the Republic of Ireland will be exempt from paying higher fees and will continue to be eligible for home fee status.

Non-EU international students

For international students from outside the UK and EU, the costs of studying in the UK are significantly greater and can often be prohibitive. For example, at Lancaster University the tuition fees for students starting in the academic year 2021–22 were £36,430 per annum, while at King's College London, international students will pay £40,800 per annum. While there is some variation in cost between universities, these fees are broadly representative of the whole of the UK.

Table 9 Tuition fees by region for courses starting in 2020

| Student's home region | Location of university or college | | | |
	England	Scotland	Wales	Northern Ireland
England	Up to £9,250	Up to £9,250	Up to £9,000	Up to £9,250
Scotland	Up to £9,250	No fee	Up to £9,000	Up to £9,250
Wales	Up to £9,250	Up to £9,250	Up to £9,000	Up to £9,250
Northern Ireland	Up to £9,250	Up to £9,250	Up to £9,000	Up to £4,395
EU & International	Variable	Variable	Variable	Variable

Financial help

There are a number of sources of financial help that are potentially available for full-time students from the UK to help cover the cost of university study. The main ones are student loans and bursaries, which are all allocated according to individual and family circumstances. It is important to apply as soon as possible through the Student Finance online service in order to prevent delay in receiving this assistance. There are different Student Finance sites to use depending on which country you are a permanent resident of. These sites contain detailed information on the help that is available and how to apply for it.

- **England:** Student Finance – www.gov.uk/studentfinance.
- **Scotland:** Student Awards Agency for Scotland (SAAS) – www.saas.gov.uk.
- **Wales:** Student Finance Wales – www.studentfinancewales.co.uk.
- **Northern Ireland:** Student Finance Northern Ireland – www.studentfinanceni.co.uk.

For the most recent figures, please check the relevant Student Finance websites regularly.

Student loans

The most common way for students to finance their studies is by taking out a student loan. If you are an eligible, full-time student, you can take out two types of loan: a loan for tuition fees and a maintenance loan to meet living costs. The tuition fees loan does not depend on your household income and is paid straight to the university to cover the full cost. You can borrow all or part of the amount required to cover your fees.

The amount of maintenance loan you are entitled to depends on several factors, including household income, where you live while you're studying and what year of study you are in. If you're living away from home, the maximum loan for English students is £9,203 for the academic year (2020–21), although it's more if you're studying in London. The maximum available is less if you're living with your parents during term time. The costs vary depending on which part of the UK you normally live in and are shown in Table 10 on page 198.

It is vital to remember when considering student loans that both the tuition fee and living expenses loans are not like loans you would get from a bank, as you only start paying it back when you have a job that pays over a certain amount. Currently these thresholds are £26,892 per annum (before deductions) for English students, £26,575 for Welsh students and £19,390 for Scottish and Northern Irish students. The repayments are then taken directly from your pay packet by your employer.

Means-tested grants

Means-tested grants for Scottish, Northern Irish and Welsh students are currently available, although this situation may change in the future. In all countries where the grant is still available, if your application for a maintenance grant is successful, the amount of loan you are entitled to will reduce accordingly.

England
While most grants have been abolished, some support may be available to certain students, for example, students with children and students with a disability.

Table 10 Maintenance loans by region

Living arrangements during term time	Maximum maintenance loan available in England	Maximum maintenance loan available in Scotland	Maximum maintenance loan available in Wales	Maximum maintenance loan available in Northern Ireland
Living at home	£7,747	£5,750	£6,885	£3,750
Living away from home and studying outside of London	£9,203	£5,750	£8,100	£4,840
Living away from home and studying in London	£12,010	£5,750	£10,124	£6,780

Wales

The Welsh Government Learning Grant (WGLG) is a grant available depending on household income. Currently, if household income is less than £18,370 per annum, the maximum amount of £8,100 is payable (not living at home outside of London). This reduces on a sliding scale to a minimum of £1,000 if income does not exceed £59,200 per annum.

Additionally, a Special Support Grant (SSG) is available for certain individuals depending on circumstances. For example, this can be paid if you are a single parent, have a disability or are in receipt of certain benefits. For the academic year 2020–21, the maximum was £5,161 per year.

Scotland

Students under the age of 25 may be entitled to the 'Young Students Bursary' (YSB), which is the equivalent of a grant. Currently, if your household income is under £20,999, you receive a maximum of £2,000. This amount then tapers to zero if you have a household income of £34,000 or over per annum. Support may also be available to certain students, for example, lone parents and students with a disability.

Northern Ireland

Special Support Grants or Maintenance Grants are available in part if household income is less than £41,065. The full grant of £3,475 is awarded if household income is £19,203 or less, and this tapers to zero up to an income of £41,065. Additional support is available to certain students, for example, lone parents and students with a disability.

In Northern Ireland, if your application for a maintenance grant is successful, the value of your maintenance loan will be reduced accordingly. However, the combined total of grant and loan will still be higher in lower-income families than higher-income ones.

NHS bursaries

Currently, students studying for medical degrees recognised by the General Medical Council may be eligible for financial assistance from the NHS for part of their course. The arrangements vary depending on your country of residence, and are set out briefly below. NB: While the rules changed for new students in some health-related fields from 1 August 2017, provision for medicine students has not been amended in the new guidelines.

England

For qualifying students, tuition fees are paid by the NHS Student Bursary scheme from the fifth year of study onwards. They will also be able to apply for a means-tested NHS bursary for living costs of up to £2,643 per year (outside London if not living with parents). The bursary award also includes access to a non-means-tested grant of £1,000. This funding information is also applicable to graduate students from their second year of study on a graduate course.

Wales

For qualifying students, tuition fees are paid in the fifth year and students can apply for a means-tested NHS Bursary (administered by Students Awards Services) from the fifth year of their course of up to £2,643 per year. In 2020–21 they would also receive a non-means-tested grant of £1,000 and a maintenance loan of up to £4,405. Graduate students on accelerated four-year programmes will be eligible for NHS funding from their second year of study onwards.

Scotland

For qualifying students, tuition fees for those studying in Scotland are paid by the Student Awards Agency Scotland (SAAS) for the duration of the course. Students can apply to the SAAS for maintenance support, which includes loans and bursaries throughout the course.

Northern Ireland

For qualifying students, income-assessed bursaries are available from the fifth year onwards. The bursaries are administered by the Department of Health, and tuition fees are also paid by the Department for the duration of the bursary. While in receipt of the bursary, students can also apply for a reduced maintenance loan from Student Finance Northern Ireland.

Further details and guidelines are available on the NHS Business Services Authority website at www.nhsbsa.nhs.uk/nhs-bursary-students.

Other sources of funding for medical students

There are various websites that will give you information on a variety of organisations that can offer scholarships, grants and bursaries that are available in addition to the NHS bursary. These include the following.

- **Armed forces bursaries/cadetships:** these are generous and may be worth considering, provided you are happy to commit to an agreed number of years working as a doctor in the Army, Navy or Air Force.
- **University bursaries:** some universities often provide bursaries for low-income students. If your household income is below £17,910 you may be eligible to receive a bursary. Some universities give bursaries to people with higher incomes. It is worth investigating this directly with your university.
- **Hardship funds:** if you are having financial problems you can apply for additional sources of funding from your institution. This is usually in the form of a bursary that doesn't have to be repaid, but might take the form of a loan. Hardship funds are administered individually by each university, so it is best to discuss directly with them.
- Students with children or responsibility for dependent adults can apply for a range of support including Childcare Grant, Parents' Learning Allowance and Child Tax Credit.
- Disabled students can apply for Disabled Students' Allowance.
- Organisations such as the Royal Medical Benevolent Fund (RMBF) (www.doctorshelp.org.uk/charity/royal-medical-benevolent-fund) can offer means-tested grants to individuals facing financial hardship due to ill health, disability or bereavement.

For more information on these, go to www.gov.uk/student-finance/extra-help and the individual university websites.

Scholarships and prizes

There are also many scholarships and prizes that are run by the many professional medical organisations. Some of the applications may require a supporting statement from a member of academic staff. Check the criteria carefully before applying.

- **British Association of Dermatologists:** offers two lots of £3,000 towards fees and living expenses for an intercalated-year project related to dermatology and skin biology. It also offers nine lots of £500 as undergraduate project grants, one £500 essay prize and three lots of £250 essay prizes.
- **Sir John Ellis Student Prizes:** students submit a description of a piece of work, survey, research or innovation in which they have been directly involved in the field of medical education. Each category awards a monetary prize and the opportunity to present their work.
- **The Genetics Society Summer Studentship scheme:** this provides funding for undergraduate students to spend their summer vacation working in a genetics laboratory in order to gain research experience:

£200 per week for up to eight weeks and £750 to contribute for costs incurred in the lab work. There are different grants available to cover any course-specific costs.

- **The Physiological Society:** the Society offers grants for students undertaking research of a physiologic nature under the supervision of a member of the society during a summer vacation or intercalated BSc year (if the student is not receiving LA or other government support).
- **The Pathological Society:** funding is offered for students wanting to intercalate a BSc in pathology who do not have LA or other government support. The Society also offers awards to fund electives and vacation studies in pathology.

Websites such as The Scholarship Hub (www.thescholarshiphub.org.uk) can also be a useful resource for finding details of available funding.

Fees for studying abroad

You should not expect the same level of financial support if you want to study overseas. If you move to the EU from 1 January 2021 to start a course, you will more than likely need to pay different fee rates compared to before Brexit. It is worth visiting individual university websites to find out the cost of studying there.

You can find out more about financial support for studying in the EU at www.gov.uk/guidance/study-in-the-european-union. There are a few grants and scholarships available through UK charities, and these are listed on the UKCISA (www.ukcisa.org.uk) and UNESCO (www.unesco.org.uk) websites.

Case study

Undeterred by the competition to study medicine in the UK, Usmaan conducted research into studying abroad. Usmaan is now is his fourth year, studying at Constanta in Romania.

'From a young age I was fascinated by medicine. The combination of ethics and science motivated me to pursue medicine as a career, as well as my interest in human anatomy. With all these things in mind, I did a lot of research into the course and undertook various work experience placements, which further fuelled my passion for studying medicine.

'We all know that getting a medical school place in the UK is difficult because it is so competitive, even if you have secured outstanding grades. I was determined that medicine was the right course for me and I didn't want to settle for anything less. My sister was already studying abroad, so I was familiar with the possibility of doing so, as

---

well as the application process and realities of studying in a different country.

'As with anything in life, studying medicine abroad has its pros and cons. That being said, I definitely feel that I made the right choice. Being far away from home makes you more independent, stronger and equips you with invaluable skills for medicine and life in general. To begin with it was hard – give yourself time to settle in and find your feet – but I quickly made friends and got into the study routine. The majority of students and staff speak English and there are many restaurants, bars and gyms to spend your leisure time. You have the option to travel home during the holidays, but social media means that it is easier than ever to stay in touch with your friends and family back home. There are many British people on the course, but it has also been great to socialise with people from lots of different backgrounds.

'The application process was fairly simple as I applied through an agent who handled most of the paperwork for me. Once my paperwork had been approved, I had to sit an entrance exam which was difficult, but a couple of months before the exam, the university provided me with practice material to get an idea of what the exam would be like. Once I had passed the exam, I received an acceptance letter confirming my place at the university, which allowed me to enrol. The agent also helped me to find an apartment, set up a new phone and gave me a tour around the area to familiarise me with it.

'Before applying to study medicine, I undertook work experience at a range of places, in charity shops, retail, pharmacies and hospitals. It's important to undertake placements in a range of areas to ensure that medicine is the right path for you. It also helped me to develop social skills, and this is important when dealing with patients further down the line and when working in a team.

'I would say my path into medicine was an unusual one as it took me longer than usual to get a place. This was purely down to my lack of commitment early on, my work ethic and my self-belief. However, I had a lot of support from my tutors at college who helped me to stay on track and pushed me to achieve the grades I needed when I was retaking my A levels, which allowed me to secure the A and A* grades I needed. My teachers were really proactive and if there was an area I was lacking in, they would pick up on this and push me in the right direction.

'Studying medicine has its ups and downs, but overall it has been a very good course. It is not easy because of the sheer amount of content, but once you get into a good study routine, managing this gets easier. For the first two years, I really enjoyed anatomy which is the foundation of any medical student's knowledge. From third year onwards, everything is clinical based, and I am in the hospital every day, putting my theoretical knowledge into practice. Once clinical placements start, you feel more like a doctor, which is particularly enjoyable. I have particularly enjoyed my orthopaedics rotation so far.

Covid-19 has restricted our clinical practice to a degree, but it has been interesting to study in this context.

'In the long run, I would like to become a consultant, but I am not sure which field I would like to specialise in just yet, as I am still to experience many more, including dermatology and gynaecology.

'I would advise prospective medical students not to lose focus. You might feel like giving up at times, but you have to persevere, especially when you are completing your A levels and everything is up in the air. You should keep the end result in the back of your mind and by taking each day as you come, you can slowly but surely work towards your goals.'

11 | Careers in medicine

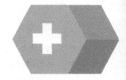

This chapter looks briefly at some of the possible careers open to prospective medics. It is of value to understand some of the avenues open to you after graduation, even if you have no firm idea about which one you want to pursue at this point.

The paths and avenues open to members of the medical profession once they graduate are too numerous to go into in detail here. As a trainee doctor nearing the end of your study, questions such as the prospect and possibility of specialisation and about where you might like to work have to be answered. The best advice we can give here is to make sure to research as much as possible, talk to people and, above all, be aware of the areas in medicine that you have enjoyed the most.

Apart from specialisations (see below), there is a wide range of areas that doctors may end up working in. Most people understand that many doctors become GPs or work in hospitals. However, there are also as many who dedicate their lives to working in areas such as public health, medical management and administration, and research.

Away from hospitals, there are careers to be made in private enterprise, for example running a consultancy business such as plastic surgery. Some doctors opt for the armed forces and others work for the police as forensic psychiatrists and forensic pathologists. Another area is education, in terms of lecturing, research and writing while working for a university. It is not uncommon to find doctors who have a portfolio of work, spending some of their time in hospitals, doing private consultancy in their own surgeries and teaching or doing research. Such a life is not only well remunerated but also highly stimulating.

First job

The training programme for doctors called Modernising Medical Careers (MMC) became fully functional in 2007. The training is part of the Certificate of Completion of Training (CCT). MMC is summarised in Figure 4 (see opposite).

In the last year of the medical degree, medical students apply for a place on the Foundation programme. The Foundation programme is designed to provide structured postgraduate training on the job and lasts two years. The job starts a few weeks after graduation from medical school. In the first few weeks there might be a short period of 'shadowing', to help new doctors get used to the job. After successful completion of the first year, they will gain registration with the GMC.

The Foundation programme job is divided into three four-month posts in the first year. These posts will typically consist of:

- four months of surgery (e.g. urology, general surgery)
- four months of another specialty (e.g. psychiatry, GP)
- four months in a medical specialty (e.g. respiratory, geriatrics).

The second year is again divided into three four-month posts, but here the focus is perhaps on a specialty or may include other jobs in shortage areas.

Final year at medical school: apply for a place on a two-year Foundation programme (www.foundationprogramme.nhs.uk)

Foundation programme starts in August
F1: three four-month placements (medicine, surgery, specialty)
F2: three four-month placements (some choice of placements)
During F2, apply for specialty registrar training (SpR) or GP registrar training
Awarded the Foundation Programme Certificate of Completion (FPCC) after successful completion of foundation training

Specialty training begins
SpR: five to eight years
GP registrar: approximately three years
After completion, receive Certificate of Completion of Training (CCT) and be eligible to go onto the SpR or GP Register

Apply for senior posts, e.g. consultant

Figure 4 MMC training structure

For more information on the application procedure, visit:

- www.foundationprogramme.nhs.uk
- www.healthcareers.nhs.uk/explore-roles/doctors

Specialisations

The MMC was introduced in 2005. It aims to provide information to doctors applying for specialty training within the NHS in England. It provides details on how to apply and the changes that occur to the recruitment and the application process. In 2012, for the first time, an agreed standardised timetable was produced for all applicants by all of the UK health departments.

Specialist training programmes typically last for five to eight years. After gaining the CCT, a doctor is then eligible to apply for a Certificate of Eligibility for Specialist Registration (CESR). Either will make you eligible for entry to the GMC's Specialist Register or GP Register.

To do this you will need to apply for postgraduate medical training programmes in the UK to the deanery or 'unit of application' directly. In this application process you will be competing for places on specialty training programmes with other doctors at similar levels of competence and experience.

For more information, visit the NHS Health Education England at http://specialtytraining.hee.nhs.uk.

Below are the major specialisations available in medicine.

- Acute Medicine
- ACCS (Acute Care Common Stem) Emergency Medicine
- Allergy
- Anaesthetics
- Anaesthetics and ACCS Anaesthetics
- Audiovestibular Medicine
- Cardiology
- Cardiothoracic Surgery
- Child and Adolescent Psychiatry
- Clinical Genetics
- Clinical Neurophysiology
- Clinical Oncology
- Clinical Pharmacology and Therapeutics
- Clinical Radiology
- Combined Infection Training
- Community Sexual and Reproductive Health
- Core Psychiatry Training
- Core Surgical Training
- Dermatology
- Diagnostic Neuropathology
- Emergency Medicine – Direct Route of Entry
- Emergency Medicine
- Endocrinology and Diabetes
- Gastroenterology
- General Practice
- General Surgery and Vascular Surgery
- Genito-urinary Medicine
- Geriatric Medicine
- Haematology
- Histopathology
- Immunology
- Intensive Care Medicine
- Internal Medicine Training and ACCS Acute Medicine
- Medical Oncology
- Medical Ophthalmology
- Metabolic Medicine
- Neurology
- Neurosurgery
- Nuclear Medicine
- Obstetrics and Gynaecology

- o Occupational Medicine
- o Ophthalmology
- o Oral and Maxillo Facial Surgery
- o Otolaryngology (Ears, Nose and Throat)
- o Paediatric and Perinatal Pathology
- o Paediatric Cardiology
- o Paediatric Surgery
- o Paediatrics
- o Palliative Medicine
- o Plastic Surgery
- o Public Health
- o Rehabilitation Medicine
- o Renal Medicine
- o Respiratory Medicine
- o Rheumatology
- o Sports and Exercise Medicine
- o Trauma and Orthopaedic Surgery
- o Urology

A few selected specialisations, briefly described, follow.

Anaesthetist

An anaesthetist is a medical doctor trained to administer anaesthesia and manage the medical care of patients before, during and after surgery. Anaesthetists are the single largest group of hospital doctors and their skills are used throughout the hospital in patient care. They have a medical background to deal with many emergency situations. They are also trained to deal with breathing, resuscitation of the heart and lungs and advanced life support.

Audiologist

Audiologists identify and assess hearing and/or balance disorders, and from this will recommend and provide appropriate rehabilitation for the patient. The main areas of work are paediatrics, adult assessment and rehabilitation, special needs groups and research and development.

Cardiologist

This is the branch of medicine that deals with disorders of the heart and blood vessels. These specialists deal with the diagnosis and treatment of heart defects, heart failure and valvular heart disease.

Dermatologist

There are over 2,000 recognised diseases of the skin but about 20 of these account for 90% of the workload. Dermatologists diagnose and treat diseases of the skin, hair and nails such as severe acne in teenagers, which is a very common reason for referral. Inflammatory skin diseases such as eczema and psoriasis are also common and without treatment can produce significant disability.

Emergency

Often referred to as the type of medicine practised in accident and emergency departments. It requires doctors to be dynamic and ready to adapt and respond at a moment's notice. Departments are led by consultants but rely on teamwork to help patients who are in an urgent condition. As you might be required to make life-saving decisions in a pressurised situation you will need a lot of confidence and belief to be in this role.

Gastroenterologist

A gastroenterologist is a medically qualified specialist who has sub-specialised in the diseases of the digestive system, which include ailments affecting all organs, from mouth to anus, along the alimentary canal. In all, a gastroenterologist undergoes a minimum of 13 years of formal classroom education and practical training before becoming a certified gastroenterologist.

General practitioner (GP)

A GP is a medical practitioner who specialises in family medicine and primary care. They are often referred to as family doctors and work in consultation clinics based in the local community.

GPs can work on their own or in a group practice with other doctors and healthcare providers. A GP treats acute and chronic illnesses and provides care and health education for all ages. They are called GPs because they look after a whole person, and this includes their mental health and physical well-being.

Gynaecologist

Gynaecologists have a broad base of knowledge and can vary their professional focus on different disorders and diseases of the female reproductive system. This includes preventive care, prenatal care and detection of sexually transmitted diseases, smear-test screening and family planning. They may choose to specialise in different areas, such as acute and chronic medical conditions, for example cervical cancer, infertility, urinary tract disorders and pregnancy and delivery.

Immunologist

Immunologists are responsible for investigating the functions of the body's immune system. They help to treat diseases such as AIDS/HIV, allergies (e.g. asthma, hay fever) and leukaemia using complex and sophisticated molecular techniques. They deal with the understanding of the processes and effects of inappropriate stimulation that are associated with allergies and transplant rejection, and may be heavily involved with research. An immunologist works within clinical and academic settings as well as with industrial research. Their role involves measuring components of the immune system, including cells, antibodies and other proteins. They develop new therapies, which involves looking at how to improve methods for treating different conditions.

Neurologist

A neurologist is trained in the diagnosis and treatment of nervous-system disorders, which includes diseases of the brain, spinal cord, nerves and muscles. They perform medical examinations of the nerves of the head and neck, muscle strength and movement, balance, ambulation and reflexes, memory, speech, language and other cognitive abilities.

Obstetrician

These are specialised doctors who deal with problems that arise during maternity care, treating any complications that develop in pregnancy and childbirth and any that arise after the birth. Some obstetricians may specialise in a particular aspect of maternity care such as maternal medicine, which involves looking after the mother's health; labour care, which involves care during the birth; and/or foetal medicine, which involves looking after the health of the unborn baby.

Paediatrician

Paediatricians deal with the growth, development and health of children from birth to adolescence. To become paediatricians, doctors must complete six years of extra training after they finish their medical training. There are general paediatricians and specialist paediatricians such as paediatric cardiologists. They work in private practices or hospitals.

Plastic surgeon

Plastic surgery is the medical and cosmetic specialty that involves the correction of form and function. There are two main types of plastic surgery: cosmetic and reconstructive.

1. Cosmetic surgery procedures alter a part of the body that the person is not satisfied with, such as breast implants or fat removal.
2. Reconstructive plastic surgery involves correcting physical birth defects, such as cleft palates, or defects that occur as a result of disease treatments, such as breast reconstruction after a mastectomy, or from accidents, such as third-degree burns after a fire.

Plastic surgery includes a variety of fields such as hand surgery, burn surgery, microsurgery and paediatric surgery.

Psychiatrist

Psychiatrists are trained in the medical, psychological and social components of mental, emotional and behavioural disorders. They specialise in the prevention, diagnosis and treatment of mental, addictive and emotional disorders such as anxiety, depression, psychosis, substance abuse and developmental disabilities. They prescribe medications, practise psychotherapy and help patients and their families cope with stress and crises. Psychiatrists often consult with primary care physicians, psychotherapists, psychologists and social workers.

Surgeon

A general surgeon is a physician who has been educated and trained in diagnosis, operative and post-operative treatment, and management of patient care. Surgery requires extensive knowledge of anatomy, emergency and intensive care, nutrition, pathology, shock and resuscitation, and wound healing. Surgeons may practise in specific fields such as general surgery, orthopaedic, neurological or vascular and many more.

Urologist

A urologist is a physician who has specialised knowledge and skills regarding problems of the male and female urinary tracts and the male reproductive organs. Extensive knowledge of internal medicine, paediatrics, gynaecology and other specialties is required by the urologist.

Some alternative careers

Armed forces

Doctors in the army are also officers, and provide medical care for soldiers and their families (https://apply.army.mod.uk/roles/army-medical-service/doctor).

Aviation medicine (also aerospace medicine)

The main role is to assess the fitness to fly of pilots, cabin crew and infirm passengers (for further information go to the website of the Faculty of Occupational Medicine www.fom.ac.uk).

Clinical forensic medical examiner (police surgeon)

Clinical forensic physicians or medical examiners spend much of their time examining people who have been arrested. Detainees either ask to see a doctor or need to be examined to see if they are fit for interview or fit to be detained (www.csofs.org).

Coroner

The coroner is responsible for inquiring into violent, sudden and unexpected, unnatural or suspicious deaths. Few are doctors, but some have qualifications in both medicine and law.

Pathologist

This job requires a variety of different specialisms, all of which combine to help form the basis of medical diagnosis. Whether it be chemical pathology, haematology, histopathology or immunology, each of which then breaks down further, there is a variety of opportunities available in clinical and lab-based research work.

Pharmaceutical medicine

Job opportunities for doctors in pharmaceutical medicine include clinical research, medical advisory positions and becoming the medical director of a company. Patient contact is limited but still possible in the clinical trials area (www.abpi.org.uk).

Prison medicine

A prison medical officer provides healthcare, usually in the form of GP clinics, to prison inmates.

Public health practitioner

Public health medicine is a specialty that deals with health at the level of a general population rather than at the level of the individual. The role can vary from responding to outbreaks of disease that need a rapid response, such as food poisoning, to the long-term planning of health-care (www.fph.org.uk).

'What is special about medicine? Everything and nothing. Everything because you have the ability to help and make a difference to people's lives. Nothing, because once you go into this career, it is your duty and part of your everyday routine. What you do matters but it is also expected. You must be serious about what you want to do because there will be many relying on you. It is tremendously rewarding and that is why anyone should go to work. In regards to the application, simply be true to you; that is the best starting place.'

Dr Emma Lumley

12 | Further information

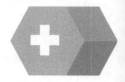

Courses

Students often have a variety of reasons for wanting to dedicate their professional lives to medicine. However, each aspiring 'future doctor' must ensure that this career choice has been an informed one. It is impossible to get a true idea of what medicine entails from just attending a course or talking to careers advisers. However, there are a number of organisations that aim to help students gain a realistic impression of medicine as a whole. Medlink is one such organisation which provides the 'Medlink' courses.

Medlink specialises in helping students in their preparation for the highly competitive medical school application process by offering day-long courses at the University of Nottingham, which are designed to give students a broader understanding of the world of medicine as well as advice on support for the application process. These courses are free. See https://medlink-uk.net to find out more.

Medic Mentor (https://medicmentor.co.uk) is another organisation that provides useful courses and resources for prospective medical students.

Publications

Careers in medicine

Being Mortal, Atul Gawande, Profile Books

Breaking & Mending: A Junior Doctor's Stories of Compassion & Burnout, Joanna Cannon, Wellcome Collection

This is Going to Hurt: Secret Diaries of a Junior Doctor, Adam Kay, Picador

Trust Me, I'm a (Junior) Doctor, Max Pemberton, Hodder

Where Does it Hurt? What the Junior Doctor Did Next, Max Pemberton, Hodder

Your Life in My Hands: A Junior Doctor's Story, Rachel Clarke, Metro Publishing

Genetics

The Blind Watchmaker, Richard Dawkins, Penguin

The Epigenetics Revolution: How Modern Biology is Rewriting Our Understanding of Genetics, Disease and Inheritance, Nessa Carey, Icon Books

The Gene: An Intimate History, Siddhartha Mukherjee, Vintage

Genome, Matt Ridley, Fourth Estate

Hacking the Code of Life: How Gene Editing will Rewrite Our Futures, Nessa Carey, Icon Books

The Immortal Life of Henrietta Lacks, Rebecca Skloot, Pan Macmillan

The Language of the Genes, Steve Jones, Flamingo

Who's Afraid of Human Cloning? Gregory E. Pence, Rowman and Littlefield

Y: The Descent of Man, Steve Jones, Abacus

Higher education entry

Getting into Oxford & Cambridge, Trotman Education

HEAP 2021: University Degree Course Offers, Trotman Education

How to Complete Your UCAS Application, Trotman Education

Medical science: general

Asimov's New Guide to Science, Isaac Asimov, Penguin

Aspirin: The Extraordinary Story of a Wonder Drug, Diarmuid Jeffreys, Bloomsbury

Don't Die Young, Dr Alice Roberts, Bloomsbury

Everything You Need to Know About Bird Flu and What You Can Do to Prepare For It, Jo Revill, Rodale

The Greatest Benefit to Mankind: A Medical History of Humanity, Roy Porter, Fontana

The Human Brain: A Guided Tour, Susan Greenfield, Phoenix

Human Instinct, Robert Winston, Bantam

The Noonday Demon: An Anatomy of Depression, Andrew Solomon, Vintage

Pain: The Science of Suffering (Maps of the Mind), Patrick Wall, Weidenfeld and Nicolson

Penicillin Man: Alexander Fleming and the Antibiotic Revolution, Kevin Brown, History Press

From Poison Arrows to Prozac: How Deadly Toxins Changed Our Lives Forever, Stanley Feldman, John Blake Publishing

A Short History of Nearly Everything, Bill Bryson, Black Swan

A User's Guide to the Brain, John Ratey, Abacus

The Vaccine Race: How Scientists Used Human Cells to Combat Killer Viruses, Meredith Wadman, Black Swan

Medical ethics

The Body Hunters: Testing New Drugs on the World's Poorest Patients, Sonia Shah, The New Press

Causing Death and Saving Lives: The Moral Problems of Abortion, Infanticide, Suicide, Euthanasia, Capital Punishment, War and Other Life-or-death Choices, Jonathan Glover, Penguin

Medical Ethics: A Very Short Introduction, Tony Hope, OUP

Medical practice

NHS Plc: The Privatisation of Our Health Care, Allyson M. Pollock, Verso

The NHS at 70, Ellen Welch, Pen and Sword History

Websites

All the medical schools have their own websites (see below) and there are numerous useful and interesting medical sites. These can be found using search engines. Particularly informative sites include the following.

- BMAT: www.admissionstesting.org/for-test-takers/bmat
- British Medical Association: www.bma.org.uk
- Department of Health: www.gov.uk/government/organisations/department-of-health-and-social-care
- General Medical Council: www.gmc-uk.org
- Student BMJ: www.student.bmj.com
- UCAT: www.ucat.ac.uk
- World Health Organisation: www.who.int

Financial advice

For information on the financial side of five to six years at medical school, see the student finance pages at www.gov.uk/student-finance. The Health Careers website (www.healthcareers.nhs.uk/career-planning/study-and-training/considering-or-university/financial-support-university) is also a useful gateway resource.

Contact details

Studying in the UK

Aberdeen
School of Medicine, Medical
Sciences and Nutrition
University of Aberdeen
Polwarth Building
Foresterhill
Aberdeen AB25 2ZD
Tel: 01224 437923
Email: medadm@abdn.ac.uk
www.abdn.ac.uk/study/under
graduate/degree-
programmes/796/A100/
medicine-5-years

Anglia Ruskin
Faculty of Medical Science
Chelmsford campus
Michael Salmon Building
Bishop Hall Lane
Chelmsford
Essex CM1 1SQ
Tel: 01245 4931319
www.anglia.ac.uk/study/under
graduate/medicine

Aston
Aston University
Birmingham B4 7ET
Tel: 0121 204 3000
Email: medicalschool@aston.
ac.uk
www2.aston.ac.uk/aston-
medical-school

Birmingham
College of Medical and Dental
Sciences
University of Birmingham
Edgbaston
Birmingham B15 2TT
Tel: 0121 414 3344
Email: mdsenquiries@contacts.
bham.ac.uk
www.birmingham.ac.uk/
university/colleges/mds/index.
aspx

Brighton and Sussex Medical School
BSMS Teaching Building
University of Sussex
Brighton BN1 9PX
Tel: 01273 606755
Email: information@sussex.ac.uk
www.bsms.ac.uk

Bristol Medical School
University of Bristol
69 St Michael's Hill
Bristol BS2 8DZ
Tel: 0117 331 1831
Email: choosebristol-ug@bristol.
ac.uk
www.bris.ac.uk/medical-school

Buckingham Medical School
The University of Buckingham
Hunter Street
Buckingham MK18 1EG
Tel: 01280 814080
Email: medicine-admissions@
buckingham.ac.uk
https://medvle.buckingham.ac.uk

Cambridge
University of Cambridge School
of Clinical Medicine
Box 111 Cambridge Biomedical
Campus
Cambridge CB2 0SP
Tel: 01223 336700
Email: admissions@cam.ac.uk
www.medschl.cam.ac.uk

Cardiff
School of Medicine
UHW Main Building
Heath Park
Cardiff CF14 4XN
Tel: 029 2087 4000
Email: medicine@cardiff.ac.uk
www.cardiff.ac.uk/medicine

Dundee
University of Dundee
Ninewells Hospital
Dundee DD1 9SY
Tel: 01382 383617
Email: asrs-medicine@dundee.ac.uk
www.dundee.ac.uk/
undergraduate/medicinek

East Anglia
Norwich Medical School
Faculty of Medicine and Health
Sciences
University of East Anglia
Norwich NR4 7TJ
Tel: 01603 591515
Email: enquiries@uea.ac.uk
www.uea.ac.uk/med

Edge Hill
Edge Hill University
St Helen's Road
Ormskirk L39 4QP
Tel: 01695 575171
Email: admissions@edgehill.ac.uk
www.edgehill.ac.uk/study/
undergraduate/medicine

Edinburgh
University of Edinburgh
The Queen's Medical Research
Institute
47 Little France Crescent
Edinburgh EH16 4TJ
Tel: 0131 242 9100
Email: medug@ed.ac.uk
www.ed.ac.uk/medicine-vet-
medicine/edinburgh-medical-
school

Exeter
University of Exeter Medical
School
St Luke's Campus
Heavitree Road
Exeter EX1 2LU
Tel: 01392 724837
Email: info.stlukes@exeter.ac.uk
http://medicine.exeter.ac.uk

Glasgow
College of Medical, Veterinary
and Life Sciences
Wolfson Medical School Building
University of Glasgow
University Avenue
Glasgow G12 8QQ
Tel: 0141 330 6216
Email: med-sch-admissions@
glasgow.ac.uk
www.gla.ac.uk/colleges/mvls

Hull York
Hull York Medical School
Allam Medical Buildings
University of Hull
Hull HU6 7RX
or
Hull York Medical School
John Hughlings Jackson Building
University of York
Heslington
York YO10 5DD
Tel: 0870 124 5500
Email: admissions@hyms.ac.uk
www.hyms.ac.uk

Imperial College London
Faculty of Medicine
Imperial College London
Level 2, Faculty Building
South Kensington Campus
London SW7 2AZ
Tel: 020 7594 7259
Email: medicine.ug.admissions@
imperial.ac.uk
www.ic.ac.uk/medicine

Keele
School of Medicine
David Weatherall Building
Keele University
Staffordshire ST5 5BG
Tel: 01782 733937
Email: medicine@keele.ac.uk
www.keele.ac.uk/medicine

King's College London
King's College London
Strand
London WC2R 2LS
Tel: 020 7836 5454
www.kcl.ac.uk/medicine

Kent and Medway
Kent and Medway Medical
School
Augustine House
Canterbury CT2 7NZ
Tel: 01227 768896
email: futuredoctors@kmms.ac.uk
https://kmms.ac.uk

Lancaster
Lancaster Medical School
Lancaster University
Lancaster LA1 4YW
Tel: 01524 594595
Email: medicine@lancaster.ac.uk
www.lancaster.ac.uk/lms

Leeds
University of Leeds
Worsley Building
Leeds LS2 9NL
Tel: 0113 343 2336
Email: ugmadmissions@leeds.
ac.uk
https://medicinehealth.leeds.
ac.uk

Leicester
University of Leicester Medical
School
George Davies Centre
Lancaster Road
Leicester LE1 7HA
Tel: 0116 252 2969/2985/3015
Email: med-admis@le.ac.uk
www2.le.ac.uk/departments/
msce/undergraduate/medicine

Lincoln
University of Lincoln
Brayford Pool
Lincoln LN6 7TS
Tel: 01522 882000
www.lincoln.ac.uk/home/course/
mdcmdcub

Liverpool
School of Medicine
MBChB Office
Cedar House
Ashton Street
Liverpool L69 3GE
Tel: 0151 795 4362
Email: mbchb@liverpool.ac.uk
www.liverpool.ac.uk/medicine

Manchester
Faculty of Biology, Medicine and
Health
University of Manchester
Oxford Road
Manchester M13 9PL
Tel: 0161 306 0211
Email: ug.medicine@manchester.
ac.uk
www.medicine.manchester.ac.uk

Newcastle
School of Medical Education
Newcastle University
Newcastle upon Tyne NE1 7RU
Tel: 0191 208 6000
Email: medic.ugadmin@ncl.ac.uk
www.ncl.ac.uk/sme/study/
undergraduate

Nottingham
Faculty of Medicine and Health
Sciences
University of Nottingham
Queen's Medical Centre
Nottingham NG7 2HA
Tel: 0115 823 0141
www.nottingham.ac.uk/mhs

Oxford
Medical Sciences Divisional
Office
University of Oxford
John Radcliffe Hospital
Headley Way
Oxford OX3 9DU
Tel: 01865 285790
Email: communications@medsci.
ox.ac.uk
www.medsci.ox.ac.uk

Plymouth
Faculty of Medicine and Dentistry
John Bull Building
Plymouth Science Park
Research Way
Plymouth PL6 8BU
Tel: 01752 600600
Email: meddent-admissions@
plymouth.ac.uk
www.plymouth.ac.uk/schools/
peninsula-medical-school

Queen's Belfast
School of Medicine, Dentistry
and Biomedical Sciences
Whitla Medical Building
97 Lisburn Road
Belfast BT9 7BL
Tel: 028 9097 2215
www.qub.ac.uk/schools/mdbs

**Queen Mary (Barts and The
London School of Medicine and
Dentistry)**
Garrod Building 4
Newark Street
Whitechapel
London E1 2AT
Tel: 020 7882 5555
Email: smdadmissions@qmul.ac.
uk
www.smd.qmul.ac.uk

St Andrews
School of Medicine
University of St Andrews
North Haugh
St Andrews KY16 9TF
Tel: 01334 463599
Email: medicine@st-andrews.ac.uk
https://medicine.st-andrews.ac.uk

St George's
St George's, University of
London
Cranmer Terrace
London SW17 0RE
Tel: 020 8672 9944
www.sgul.ac.uk

Sheffield
The Medical School
University of Sheffield
Beech Hill Road
Sheffield S10 2RX
Tel: 0114 222 5522
Email: med-school@sheffield.ac.uk
www.shef.ac.uk/medicine

Southampton
Faculty of Medicine
University of Southampton
12 University Road
Southampton SO17 1BJ
Tel: 023 8059 5571
Email: ugapply.fm@southampton.
ac.uk
www.southampton.ac.uk/
medicine

Sunderland
The University of Sunderland
Edinburgh Building
City Campus Chester Road
Sunderland SR1 3SD
Tel: 0191 515 2000
Email: student.helpline@sunder-
land.ac.uk
www.sunderland.ac.uk/about/
school-of-medicine

Swansea
Swansea University Medical
School
Grove Building
Institute of Life Science
Swansea SA2 8QA
Tel: 01792 602697
Email: studt@swansea.ac.uk
www.swan.ac.uk/medicine

University College London
UCL Medical School
74 Huntley Street
London WC1E 6BT
Tel: 020 3108 8235/7674/6185
Email: medicaladmissions@ucl.
ac.uk
www.ucl.ac.uk/medicalschool

UCLAN
University of Central Lancashire
Fylde Road
Preston PR1 2HE
Tel: 01772 210210
Email: cenquiries@uclan.ac.uk
www.uclan.ac.uk/courses/
bachelor_medicine_bachelor_sur-
gery.php

Warwick
Warwick Medical School
University of Warwick
Coventry CV4 7HL
Tel: 02476 574880
Email: wmsinfo@warwick.ac.uk
www2.warwick.ac.uk/fac/med

Volunteering

British Red Cross
44 Moorfields
London EC2Y 9AL
Tel: 0344 871 1111
Email: contactus@redcross.org.uk
www.redcross.org.uk/Get-involved/Volunteer

Do-it (database for volunteering placements)
www.do-it.org.uk

NHS Volunteering
www.england.nhs.uk/participation/get-involved/volunteering

Positive East (HIV/AIDS volunteering)
159 Mile End Road
London E1 4AQ
Tel: 020 7791 2855
Email: talktome@positiveeast.org.uk
www.positiveeast.org.uk

vInspired
Unit 3, 9 Albert Embankment
London SE1 7SP
Tel: 020 7960 7000
Email: info@vinspired.com
https://vinspired.com

Volunteering Matters
The Levy Centre
18–24 Lower Clapton Road
London E5 0PD
Tel: 020 3780 5870
https://volunteeringmatters.org.uk

It is worthwhile contacting your local county or borough council and local hospital to find out what volunteering opportunities it has, for example, in hospitals, care homes or schools (all of which will require criminal record DBS checks).

Health careers

www.healthcareers.nhs.uk/career-planning/improving-your-chances/gaining-experience

Working abroad

www.workingabroad.com/project-finder
www.globalpremeds.com/gap-medics

Tables

Table 11 Medical school admissions policies for 2021–22

Institution	Usual offer	Required A level subjects	Retakes considered	Minimum GCSE requirements
Aberdeen	AAA (IB 36 points with 3 at HL, Grade 6)	Chemistry plus one from Biology, Maths and Physics	Not usually, but may consider if there were verifiable serious personal difficulties at the time of the first sitting	Grade 6 in English Language and Maths required. Biology and Physics recommended. Combination of grades 6–9 are expected
Anglia Ruskin	AAA (IB min 36 points, 6,6,6 at HL Biology and/or Chemistry, plus one other science and Maths or English)	Chemistry or Biology and one of Biology, Chemistry, Maths or Physics	Yes, resit grades of AAA will be accepted if taken within two academic years prior to the time of application	5 GCSEs at grade 9–6 (A*–7), including English Language, Maths and 2 sciences
Aston	AAA–ABB (if contextual factors are met) (IB 36 points, with 6,6,6 at HL including Chemistry and Biology)	Biology and Chemistry	Yes, but only one resit attempt considered; reasons for resitting must be outlined in the UCAS reference	Minimum of 7 GCSEs at 6/B or above. Must include English Language, Maths, Chemistry, Biology or Double Science
Birmingham	AAA (IB 32 points, with HL 6,6,6 including Biology, Chemistry and 1 other)	Biology and Chemistry	Only if very serious life events that occurred at an important stage in education. Repeat applications are not permitted	At least 5 subjects, including English Language, Maths, Biology and Chemistry, at grade 6/B
Brighton and Sussex	AAA (IB 36 points, with 6, 6 in Biology and Chemistry)	Biology and Chemistry	Yes, if narrowly missed by one grade in one subject or if have final grades of AAA after 3 years	Grade6/B or above in Maths and English Language or Literature
Bristol	AAA (IB 36 points with 18 points at HL including 6s in Chemistry and one of Biology, Physics or Maths)	Chemistry and either Biology, Physics or Maths	Yes	7/A in Maths, 4/C in English Language
Brunel (non-UK students only)	AAB (IB 33 points, 6, 5 in Chemistry or Biology, plus one from Chemistry, Biology, Physics or Maths)	Chemistry or Biology plus one from Chemistry, Biology, Physics or Maths	Considered on a case-by-case basis where there have been genuine extenuating circumstances	5 subjects at 4/C to include English Language and Maths
Buckingham	AAB (IB 34 points, with 6, 6 in Biology and Chemistry)	Chemistry and one from Maths or Biology	Yes	5/C in English and Maths, 6/B in Biology if not offered at A level
Cambridge	A*A*A (IB 40–42 with HL 7,7,6)	Chemistry and one from Biology Physics or Maths, although 3 sciences/maths are preferred	In extenuating circumstances	None

***Note:** Details were correct when going to press – check websites for updated information.*

Table 11 Continued

Institution	Usual offer	Required A level subjects	Retakes considered	Minimum GCSE requirements
Central Lancashire (UCLAN)	AAB	At least 2 science subjects, including Chemistry, and a third academic subject	No	English Language to grade 6/B
Cardiff	AAA (IB 36 with 19 at HL including 6 in Biology and Chemistry)	Biology and Chemistry	Only in exceptional circumstances and if previously applied to Cardiff	English Language at 6/B and 8 GCSEs at 6/B including Biology, Chemistry and Maths
Dundee	AAA–ABB (IB 37 including 6,6,6 at HL including HL Chemistry and another science)	Chemistry and one from Biology, Physics or Maths	No	Biology, Maths and English at 6/B if not studied at A level
East Anglia	AAA (IB 36, 6,6,6 in all HL subjects including Biology or Chemistry)	Biology or Chemistry	Yes (ABB or AAC or equivalent from first sitting); an A* will form part of the offer	6 GCSEs at 7/A or above to include Maths and 2 Sciences, with English Language at 6/B
Edge Hill	AAA (IB 36, with 6 in Biology and Chemistry and one other subject)	Biology and Chemistry	Yes	At least 5 GCSEs at 6/B to include Biology, Chemistry, English Language and Maths
Edinburgh	AAA (IB 37, with HL 6,6,7)	Chemistry and one of Biology, Maths or Physics	In extenuating circumstances (evidence must be verified prior to UCAS application)	6/B in Biology, Chemistry, English, Maths
Exeter	AAA (IB36 with 6,6,6 overall to include Biology and Chemistry at HL)	Chemistry and Biology	Yes	4/C in English Language
Glasgow	AAA (IB 38, with 6 in HL Biology and Chemistry SL Physics or Maths)	Chemistry and Biology, Maths or Physics	In extenuating circumstances	Maths and English Language at 6/B or above
Hull York	AAA (IB 36,with HL 6,6,5 including Biology and Chemistry)	Biology and Chemistry	Yes, if achieved BBB at first sitting and taken in one extra year	6 at A*/9 to C/4
Imperial	A*AA–AAA (IB 38, with 6 in HL Biology and Chemistry)	Chemistry and Biology	Not usually, but contact the admissions team to discuss specific circumstances	6/B in English Language
Keele	A*AA (IB 35, with 6 in all HL subjects)	Biology or Chemistry and another science (Biology, Chemistry, Physics or Maths)	Only if applying after total of three years of A level study with achieved grades	5 A/7 with Maths, English Language and Science at B/6 or above

Table 11 Continued

Institution	Usual offer	Required A level subjects	Retakes considered	Minimum GCSE requirements
Kent and Medway	AAB (IB 34, with 6 in Biology or Chemistry and one of Biology, Chemistry, Maths, Physics or Psychology at 6)	Chemistry or Biology, plus one of Chemistry, Biology, Maths Physics, Psychology or Computer Science	Only if there is extenuating circumstances	At least 5 at 9–6/A*–B including English Language, Maths, Biology, Chemistry and Physics
King's	A*AA (IB 35, with 7,6,6 in Biology and Chemistry)	Biology and Chemistry	Only if there are serious mitigating circumstances	B/6 in English and Maths
Lancaster	AAA–AAB (IB 36, with HL 6,6,6 including 6 in any 2 of Biology, Chemistry and Psychology). 6 in Biology and Chemistry)	Two of Biology, Chemistry and Psychology	Yes, if achieved ABB at first attempt	Eight subjects, including 6/B in Biology, Chemistry, Physics, English Language and Maths
Leeds	AAA (IB 34, 3 HL grade 5, one must be Biology or Chemistry)	Chemistry or Biology (if no Chemistry, Physics or Maths must be taken)	Only in extenuating circumstances	6 at minimum grade 4/C including Chemistry and Biology, English Language and Maths
Leicester	AAA (IB 34, with 6 in all HL subjects, including Chemistry or Biology plus one from Biology, Chemistry, Maths, Physics or Psychology)	Chemistry or Biology, and one from Biology, Chemistry, Maths, Physics or Psychology	Only if achieved AAB or AEB in first attempt	6/B in English Language, Maths, Biology and Chemistry
Lincoln	AAA (IB 36, with 6 in all HL subjects including Biology and Chemistry)	Biology and Chemistry	No	Six GCSEs at 7/A including Biology, Chemistry, Physics and Maths, plus English Language at 6/B
Liverpool	AAA (IB 36, with 6 in HL Chemistry with either Biology, Physics or Maths)	Chemistry, with either Biology, Physics or Mathematics	Yes, with AEB at first sitting	9 GCSEs including Biology, Chemistry, Physics, English Language and Maths. Score must be better than 15 for best 9 sucjects, with A*/A = 2 and B = 1.
Manchester	AAA (IB 37, with HL 7,6,6 in Chemistry or Biology and one from Chemistry, Biology, Physics, Psychology, Maths)	Chemistry or Bioogy and one from Chemistry, Biology, Physics, Psychology, Maths and Further Maths	Yes, if no lower than BBB in first sitting. Required grades will be A*AA	At least 7 at 7/A or 8/A*, English Language, Maths and 2 sciences at 6/B or above
Newcastle	AAA (IB 38)	None listed	In extenuating circumstances	None listed

Note: Details were correct when going to press – check websites for updated information.

Table 11 Continued

Institution	Usual offer	Required A level subjects	Retakes considered	Minimum GCSE requirements
Nottingham	AAA (IB 36, with 6 in HL subjects inc. Biology and Chemistry)	Biology and Chemistry	Yes, with ABB at first sitting with the A in Biology or Chemistry	6 GCSEs at 7/A A to include Chemistry, Biology, Physics and Maths, plus English Language at 6/B
Oxford	A*AA (IB 39 with HL 7, 6, 6)	Chemistry and one from Biology, Physics, Maths or Further Maths	Potentially, but contact university for specific advice	No formal GCSE requirements
Plymouth	A*AA–AAB (IB 36–38 with 6 in HL Biology plus one further science from Chemistry, Maths, Physics and Psychology)	Biology and one from Chemistry, Physics, Maths and Psychology	Yes if ABB at first attempt	7 at 9-4/A*–C, including English Language, Maths and 2 sciences
Queen Mary, University of London	A*AA (38 points with 6,6,6 in HL subjects including Biology or Chemistry and a second science or Maths	Biology or Chemistry plus a second science from Chemistry, Biology, Physics and Maths	Only with serious extenuating circumstances if the student is protected under the Equality and Diversity Act	English Language, Biology, Chemistry and Maths at 7,7,6,6,6 or A,A,A,B,B
Queen's Belfast	A*AA (IB 36, with 6,6,6 in HL subjects)	Chemistry and Biology	If previously accepted Queen's offer and missed by 1 grade (A*AB at first attempt)	GCSE scored on best 9 subjects, so high grades will be advantageous. Maths and Physics at 4/C if not offered at AS or A level
St Andrews	AAA (IB 38 with HL 6,6,6)	Chemistry and one from Biology, Physics or Maths	In extenuating circumstances if close to meeting entry requirements	5 7/A grades
St George's	A*AA–AAA (IB 36 with 18 points at HL and 6 in Biology and Chemistry)	Biology and Chemistry	No	5 GCSEs at 6/B or above, including English Language, Maths and Science
Sheffield	AAA (IB 36 with 6 in HL subjects including Chemistry or Biology or one other science subject)	Chemistry or Biology and one other from Chemistry, Biology, Psychology or Maths	Yes	At least 5 7/A grades including at least 6/B in Maths, English Language and the sciences
Southampton	AAA (IB 36 with 6 in HL subjects including Biology and one other science)	Biology and one from Chemistry, Physics, Psychology, Sociology, Environmental Studies or Geography	Yes	7 GCSEs at 6/B including Maths, Biology Chemistry and English Language
Sunderland	AAA (IB 35, 6,6,6 in HL subjects to include Chemistry or Biology)	Biology or Chemistry and a second science from Biology, Chemistry, Maths	Yes	5 GCSEs at 7/A with 6/B in English language, Maths, Biology, Chemistry and Physics
UCL	A*AA (IB 39, with 19 in HL subjects, with 6 in Biology and Chemistry)	Biology and Chemistry	No	6/B in English Language and Maths: UK students also need 5/C in a foreign language

Note: Details were correct when going to press – check websites for updated information.

Table 12 Medical school interview and written test policies for 2021–22

Institution	Type and typical length (minutes)	Number on the panel (if applicable)	Pre-admissions test	Information on how UCAT is used
Aberdeen	MMI, 60 minutes	n/a	UCAT	UCAT cut-off score is not used. No strict ranking of scores. In 2020, interviewed applicants ranged between scores of 2420 and 3510.
Anglia Ruskin	MMI	n/a	UCAT	Applicants are ranked according to score.
Aston	MMI	n/a	UCAT	Considered alongside the other required qualifications.
Birmingham	MMI	n/a	UCAT	No minimum cut-off, but in 2020, the threshold score was 2640.
Brighton and Sussex	MMI	n/a	BMAT	n/a
Bristol	MMI	n/a	UCAT	No set cut-off score, but combined score of all subtests except SJT is used to select for interview.
Buckingham	MMI	n/a	None	n/a
Cambridge	Panel, 2 interviews each 25-30 minutes	At least 1 current practitioner	BMAT	n/a
Cardiff	MMI	n/a	UCAT/ GAMSAT	Used holistically as part of the selection process, but no strict cut-off.
Dundee	MMI	n/a	UCAT	No minimum cut-off score.
East Anglia	MMI	n/a	UCAT	No cut-off score, but a high score is advantageous.
Edge Hill	MMI	n/a	UCAT	Scores are ranked, and there is a cut-off to select for interview. SJT band 4 is immediately rejected.
Edinburgh	MMI (interviews only for graduate and mature applicants)	n/a	UCAT	All scores accepted, no minimum requirement but total UCAT score and SJT used with academic profile to rank applicants.
Exeter	MMI	n/a	UCAT/ GAMSAT	Applicants sorted according to academic profile and UCAT overall score to determine if interviewed.
Glasgow	Panel, 2 interviews lasting a total of 30 minutes	Each panel consists of 2 interviewers	UCAT	UCAT score is used together with academic profile to select for interview.

Table 12 Continued

Institution	Type and typical length (minutes)	Number on the panel (if applicable)	Pre-admissions test	Information on how UCAT is used
Hull-York	MMI	n/a	UCAT	Total score plus SJT band is given a points score to be used alongside GCSE results and contextual data.
Imperial	MMI	n/a	BMAT	n/a
Keele	MMI	n/a	UCAT (home applications) BMAT (international applications)	Used to separate candidates in borderline cases.
Kent Medway	MMI	n/a	UCAT	There is a minimum threshold for total UCAT score, although it is described as 'generous'.
King's	MMI	n/a	UCAT	The overall average score and SJT are taken into account when shortlisting candidates, but there is no cut-off score.
Lancaster	MMI	n/a	BMAT	n/a
Leeds	MMI	n/a	BMAT	n/a
Leicester	MMI, 60 minutes	n/a	UCAT	No minimum cut-off, but but performance is scored along with academic performce. SJT band 4 are rejected immediately.
Lincoln	MMI	n/a	UCAT	No fixed UCAT threshold.
Liverpool	MMI	n/a	UCAT/ GAMSAT	Scores are ranked and top scoring applicants are invited to interview. SJT band 4 is rejected.
Manchester	MMI	n/a	UCAT	If score is in top third of all results nationally, you will be invited to interview if you meet the other criteria. However, lower scores will be considered if rest of profile is strong.
Newcastle	Newcastle MMI (Home) Panel (International)	2	UCAT	Students above threshold score who meet academic require-ments are invited to interview. 2020 threshold was 2730.
Nottingham	MMI	n/a	UCAT	UCAT score is added to GCSE score, and combined score is used for interview selection. There is no fixed threshold.
Oxford	Panel (interviews at two colleges)	At least 2 academics at each college	BMAT	n/a

Table 12 Continued

Institution	Type and typical length (minutes)	Number on the panel (if applicable)	Pre-admissions test	Information on how UCAT is used
Plymouth	MMI	n/a	UCAT/GAM-SAT	Score must be above threshold. For 2021 entry, this was 2400.
Queen Mary	Panel, 15 to 20 minutes	2–4	UCAT	Score given a 50:50 weighting with academic profile. If score is below third decile nationally, application is rejected.
Queen's Belfast	MMI	n/a	UCAT	Score used alongside GCSE profile to rank for interview.
ScotGEM (Graduate only)	MMI	n/a	GAMSAT	n/a
Sheffield	MMI	n/a	UCAT	Scores below the current threshold of 2420 are rejected. All other scores are ranked to determine who is invited to interview.
Southampton	Selection day	n/a	UCAT	Scores ranked to determine who is invited to selection day.
St Andrews	MMI	n/a	UCAT	If application has met academic criteria, UCAT score is then ranked, with approximately top 400 invited to interview.
St George's	MMI	n/a	UCAT	Thresholds for the individual sections and overall score must be met. In 2020, this was 500 in each section and 2480 overall.
Sunderland	MMI and a maths test	n/a	UCAT	UCAT score must be within top 8 deciles of the cohort, with SJT band 1–3.
Swansea (Graduate only)	Panel (2 interviews with 30-minute written test)	2	GAMSAT	n/a
UCL	Panel	n/a	BMAT	n/a
UCLAN	MMI	n/a	None	n/a
Warwick (Graduate only)	MMI	n/a	UCAT	First round of selection rejects applicants with verbal reasoning scores below the UCAT average. The rest of the sections are then scored to produce an overall score. In 2019, a total of 2570 was needed to be invited to interview.

MMIs are multiple mini interviews, a series of small interviews or tasks the candidate has to complete. Their content varies with the medical school that carries them out. See the individual websites for more details. Source: University websites and Medical Schools Council website; correct at time of going to print.

Glossary

AIDS (acquired immune deficiency syndrome)
AIDS is a disease that affects the immune system, lowering the body's resistance to infection. The disease is caused by the human immuno-deficiency virus (HIV).

BHA (British Humanist Association)
The association acting for those who are non-religious who seek to live ethical lives on the basis of reason and humanity.

BMA (British Medical Association)
The professional medical association and trade union for doctors and medical students.

BMAT (BioMedical Admissions Test)
An admissions test required by certain universities. See Table 6 on page 78 for a list of universities that require this test.

BMI (body mass index)
Indicates whether someone is overweight or underweight, based on their weight and height.

CBL (Case-based learning)
The medical training that some medical schools use that is more case led, based on clinical examples, than the more problem-based learning courses.

CSP (Chartered Society of Physiotherapists)
Professional, educational and trade union body for the UK's physiother-apy workforce.

GAMSAT (Graduate Medical School Admissions Test)
A test introduced in 1999 by some universities to aid in the selection of candidates who already have degrees.

GEP (Graduate Entry Programme)
A four-year programme offered by universities for students who already have a degree, as opposed to the traditional five-year programme.

GMC (General Medical Council)
The governing body that protects, promotes and maintains the health and safety of the public by ensuring proper standards in the practice of medicine.

Integrated courses
Those where basic medical sciences are taught concurrently with clinical studies. Thus, this style is a compromise between a traditional course and a PBL course.

Intercalated degree
An intercalated degree is a one-year course of study after the pre-clinical years to attain a further degree, e.g. in biochemistry or anatomy.

MB (Bachelor of Medicine)
One of the three degrees that can be awarded by medical schools to students after four or five years of academic study.

MBBS (Bachelor of Medicine and Surgery)
One of the three degrees that can be awarded by medical schools to students after four or five years of academic study.

MBChB
Some medical schools award this degree instead of the MBBS. This depends on the medical school.

MMR (measles, mumps and rubella)
A vaccination given to young children around the age of one.

MRI (magnetic resonance imaging)
A medical imaging technique used in radiology to visualise detailed internal structures of the body.

MRSA (methicillin-resistant *Staphylococcus aureus*)
A bacterium responsible for several difficult-to-treat infections in humans. It is also called multidrug-resistant bacteria.

NICE (National Institute for Health and Care Excellence)
NICE sets standards for quality healthcare and produces guidance on medicines, treatments and procedures.

PBL (problem-based learning)
The medical training that some medical schools use and is a more patient-oriented approach than the more traditional lecture styles.

Personal statement
The written document provided by the candidate about themselves which is sent with the university application to the medical schools.

PLAB
The Professional Linguistic and Assessment Board sets a test for assessing eligibility for students entering the UK to practise medicine having studied abroad.

Student BMJ
A publication produced for medical students.

Traditional courses
Longer established and following a lecture-based style, using didactic methods. The majority of these courses are subject-based ones, where lectures are the most appropriate way of delivering the information.

UCAS (Universities and Colleges Admissions Service)
The central body through which students apply to medical school or any higher education institution.

UCAS codes
The identifying letters and numbers of the various university courses. These are vital when making your application. Medical courses range from A100 to A104 depending on previous experience (e.g. A levels, degree, etc.).

UCAT (University Clinical Aptitude Test)
An application test that certain medical schools require students to sit before accepting them onto the course. See Table 4 on page 61 for a list of which universities require this test.

WHO (World Health Organization)
A specialised agency of the United Nations that acts as a coordinating authority on international public health.

Work experience
Voluntary work (normally) organised before you apply to medical school which is described in your personal statement. This is a vital component of your application.